Genetic Disorders

Peggy J. Parks

Diseases and Disorders

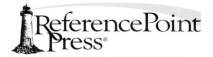

ReferencePoint
Press®

San Diego, CA

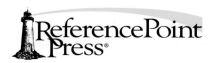

About the Author:
Peggy J. Parks holds a bachelor of science degree from Aquinas College in Grand Rapids, Michigan, where she graduated magna cum laude. She has written more than 80 nonfiction educational books for children and young adults, as well as published a cookbook called *Welcome Home: Recipes, Memories, and Traditions from the Heart*. Parks lives in Muskegon, Michigan, a town that she says inspires her writing because of its location on the shores of Lake Michigan.

For more information, contact:
ReferencePoint Press, Inc.
PO Box 27779
San Diego, CA 92198
www. ReferencePointPress.com

Picture credits:
Cover: iStockphoto.com
Maury Aaseng: 31–33, 46–48, 62–65, 77–79
AP Images: 10, 15

LIBRARY OF CONGRESS CATALOGING-IN-PUBLICATION DATA

Parks, Peggy J., 1951–
    Genetic disorders / by Peggy J. Parks.
        p. cm. — (Compact research series)
    Includes bibliographical references and index.
    ISBN-13: 978-1-60152-096-8 (hardback)
    ISBN-10: 1-60152-096-4 (hardback)
    1. Genetic disorders—Juvenile literature. I. Title.
    RB155.5.P37 2009
    616'.042—dc22

                                                                    2009025065

Contents

Foreword

66 **Where is the knowledge we have lost in information?** 99

—T.S. Eliot, "The Rock."

As modern civilization continues to evolve, its ability to create, store, distribute, and access information expands exponentially. The explosion of information from all media continues to increase at a phenomenal rate. By 2020 some experts predict the worldwide information base will double every 73 days. While access to diverse sources of information and perspectives is paramount to any democratic society, information alone cannot help people gain knowledge and understanding. Information must be organized and presented clearly and succinctly in order to be understood. The challenge in the digital age becomes not the creation of information, but how best to sort, organize, enhance, and present information.

ReferencePoint Press developed the *Compact Research* series with this challenge of the information age in mind. More than any other subject area today, researching current issues can yield vast, diverse, and unqualified information that can be intimidating and overwhelming for even the most advanced and motivated researcher. The *Compact Research* series offers a compact, relevant, intelligent, and conveniently organized collection of information covering a variety of current topics ranging from illegal immigration and deforestation to diseases such as anorexia and meningitis.

The series focuses on three types of information: objective single-author narratives, opinion-based primary source quotations, and facts and statistics. The clearly written objective narratives provide context and reliable background information. Primary source quotes are carefully selected and cited, exposing the reader to differing points of view. And facts and statistics sections aid the reader in evaluating perspectives. Presenting these key types of information creates a richer, more balanced learning experience.

For better understanding and convenience, the series enhances information by organizing it into narrower topics and adding design features that make it easy for a reader to identify desired content. For example, in *Compact Research: Illegal Immigration*, a chapter covering the economic impact of illegal immigration has an objective narrative explaining the various ways the economy is impacted, a balanced section of numerous primary source quotes on the topic, followed by facts and full-color illustrations to encourage evaluation of contrasting perspectives.

The ancient Roman philosopher Lucius Annaeus Seneca wrote, "It is quality rather than quantity that matters." More than just a collection of content, the *Compact Research* series is simply committed to creating, finding, organizing, and presenting the most relevant and appropriate amount of information on a current topic in a user-friendly style that invites, intrigues, and fosters understanding.

Genetic Disorders at a Glance

Genetic Disorders Defined

There are thousands of genetic disorders, and they are defined as conditions in which an individual's genetic makeup has been altered in some way.

Types of Genetic Disorders

The three main categories are single-gene disorders, chromosome disorders, and multifactorial inheritance disorders. What they all have in common is that they result from genetic abnormalities.

Prevalence

The prevalence of genetic disorders varies widely depending on the type. For instance, at least 1.3 million people in the United States suffer from congenital heart defects, while 1.5 million Americans have Parkinson's disease, 500,000 suffer from multiple sclerosis, and an estimated 30,000 have Huntington's disease.

Symptoms

When symptoms appear depends on the type of disorder. For instance, babies born with Down syndrome or dwarfism can usually be diagnosed at birth, while those with hereditary forms of cancer, heart disease, and Alzheimer's disease may not be diagnosed until decades later.

Causes

Genetic disorders occur as the result of defective genes that are passed to a child from the mother, the father, or both. Multifactorial genetic disorders are the result of a combination of genetic and environmental factors.

Diagnosis and Treatment

Genetic disorders can be determined through a variety of tests, from blood tests to ultrasounds and X-rays. Some disorders can be successfully treated, while for others, such as Down syndrome, Tay-Sachs disease, and Huntington's disease, there is no treatment.

Genetic Testing

Genetic testing can show someone's risk for developing a variety of hereditary diseases. Tests can also show whether someone is a carrier of abnormal genes or whether a fetus likely has a genetic disorder.

Controversial Issues

Genetic testing is controversial because test results can cause fear in those who learn that they will develop an incurable disease but can do nothing to stop it. Prenatal testing is controversial because if a fetus is believed to have a genetic disorder, this often leads to abortion.

Progress Toward a Cure

Because genetic disorders are so diverse, with so many contributors, there is no way for scientists to develop one cure. Research has led to a multitude of treatments that have vastly improved the lives of people who suffer from many genetic disorders, and in some cases the patients are considered cured.

Overview

> **A genetic disorder is a disease that is caused by an abnormality in an individual's DNA. Abnormalities can range from a small mutation in a single gene to the addition or subtraction of an entire chromosome or set of chromosomes.**
>
> —Genetic Science Learning Center, a science and health education program at the University of Utah.

> **Simply having problem genes is only half the story because many illnesses develop from a mix of high-risk genes and environmental factors.**
>
> —Linda Nicholson, a certified genetics counselor at Arcadia University in Pennsylvania.

Jeffrey Carroll knows that he will eventually develop Huntington's disease, a devastating genetic disorder for which there is no treatment or cure. After both his grandmother and mother died from the disease, Carroll underwent genetic testing and found that he, too, carried the Huntington's gene. "It is the most profound thing," he says. "You know how you probably are going to die. You watched somebody you love die the exact same way." It was extremely painful for Carroll to watch his mother slowly waste away until she was no longer able to walk, talk, think, or even swallow. What began with small muscle ticks and mild tremors escalated into shaking and thrashing that was so violent, she had to be placed on floor mats at the nursing home where she was being cared for. "Killing you is not the cruel part of this disease," Carroll says. "It destroys your personality and turns you into an object of horror for your family. Even if they love you, nobody can watch it and not be horrified."[1]

Once Carroll received his own test result, he decided to turn it into something positive, rather than spending his time being terrified of what was to come. He is a scientist at Canada's biggest laboratory for the study of Huntington's disease, and he is devoting his career to the search for a cure. Yet even though Carroll is passionate about his work, he is always aware that symptoms will begin and the disease will claim his life. "I know how awful it is going to be," he says. "It's the only thing, I often think, that makes me different . . . the knowledge that I am one of them, that I am going to die. I know how I am going to die."[2]

The Human Genome

Before one can understand genetic disorders, it is important to have an understanding of the human body's genetic makeup, known as the genome. The body is composed of trillions of cells, the building blocks of all living things. Within cells that have a nucleus (such as white blood cells) is deoxyribonucleic acid (DNA), the "blueprint" of life. DNA molecules are packed into large, complex, threadlike structures known as chromosomes. Genes (of which there are more than 20,000 in the human body) are the basic unit of heredity and are composed of DNA. An article on the Web site Science Clarified explains the important role played by genes: "A vast range of human characteristics, from eye and hair color to musical and literary talents, are controlled by genes. To say that a person has red hair color, for example, is simply to say that that person's body contains genes that tell hair cells how to make red hair."[3]

> " Before one can understand genetic disorders, it is important to have an understanding of the human body's genetic makeup, known as the genome. "

What Are Genetic Disorders?

A genetic disorder is a condition in which an individual's genetic makeup has been altered in some way. For instance, people with Hunter syndrome are missing an enzyme that is used to break down cellular waste products in the body, while those with Down syndrome have inherited chromosomal abnormalities from one or both parents. People who have cystic fibrosis have abnormalities in the CFTR gene, which makes a protein that controls the movement of salt and water in and out of the body's cells. BRCA1 and BRCA2 are tumor suppressor genes; when mutations occur (due to heredity), the genes no longer suppress abnormal growth, and this can lead to breast and ovarian cancer.

Types of Genetic Disorders

Thousands of diseases and disorders trace back to genetics. The three main categories are: single-gene disorders, chromosome disorders, and multifactorial inheritance disorders. Single-gene disorders, including cystic fibrosis, sickle-cell anemia, and Huntington's disease, are the result of a mutation in a single gene. Chromosome disorders such as Down syndrome involve

A young woman from Idaho adjusts the device that allows her to inhale medicine used to treat cystic fibrosis, an inherited disease that clogs the lungs, intestines, and pancreas with thick mucus. The disease has no cure, but modern medicines allow patients to live longer than in the past.

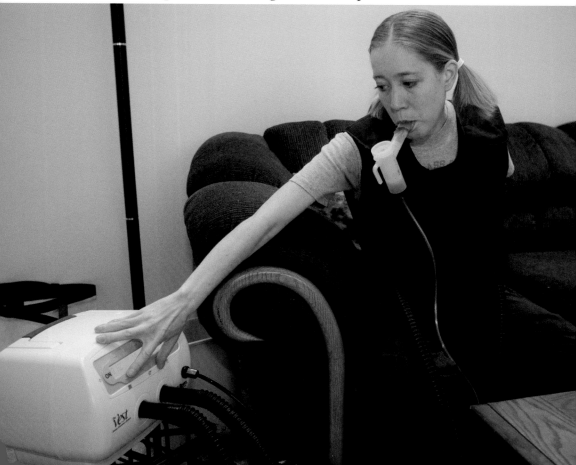

an excess or deficiency in the genes located on chromosomes or structural changes within chromosomes. Multifactorial inheritance disorders such as some types of heart disease and cancer, multiple sclerosis, and Alzheimer's disease, result from a combination of genetic and environmental factors.

Although many genetic disorders have devastating effects and in some cases lead to death, some are not life threatening but can be frustrating for those who suffer from them. One example of this is color blindness. According to the National Institutes of Health, the most common form of color blindness is red-green vision defects, in which affected people have problems distinguishing between shades of red and green. Those with blue-yellow color vision defects have difficulty distinguishing shades of blue and yellow. People who suffer from an extremely rare form of color blindness known as achromatopsia cannot perceive any colors and see only black, white, and shades of gray. In the United States, only about 1 in 40,000 children are born with achromatopsia. In other areas of the world, especially those where marriages between relatives are common practice, the disorder is much more prevalent. On the tiny Pacific island of Pingelap, as much as 10 percent of the native population has achromatopsia. It is so prevalent that Pingelap is often referred to as the "Island of the Color Blind."

> **People who suffer from an extremely rare form of color blindness known as achromatopsia cannot perceive any colors and see only black, white, and shades of gray.**

Symptoms of Genetic Disorders

Whether the characteristics of genetic disorders are obvious immediately at birth or not until later depends on the type. For instance, infants who have an extremely rare genetic disorder known as Smith-Lemli-Opitz syndrome are born with severe physical abnormalities such as microcephaly (small head), extra fingers or toes, webbing between the second and third toes, and/or drooping eyelids. Babies born with Tay-Sachs, a rapidly progressing nervous system disease, appear to be perfectly healthy and normal at birth. Symptoms of Tay-Sachs, including noticeable behavior changes, seizures, slow body growth, and delayed mental and social skills, often do not show up until three to six months of age. Children born with Hunter syndrome may go for years without being diagnosed. Those with late onset Hunter syndrome often do not develop symptoms until they are past 10 years old and it becomes apparent that they have abnormal bone size or shape, joint stiffness, hearing loss, and poor peripheral vision.

Hereditary forms of cancer may not show up for decades, when a person notices an unusual growth, abnormal bleeding, or other suspicious physical problems. Babies who are born with congenital heart defects may develop a bluish tinge around the lips and on the fingers, which is a sign that the body is not receiving enough oxygen. But many children and adults who have the disorder do not realize that anything is wrong until later in life when they experience chest pains or have a heart attack. The same is true of hereditary forms of Alzheimer's disease (early onset types), in which the majority of symptoms do not become apparent until people are in their forties or fifties. Alzheimer's is usually first noticeable when someone experiences confusion and memory loss. As the disease progresses and the brain continues to waste away, the symptoms worsen, and the person will die from Alzheimer's-related complications, usually infection or pneumonia.

> " **Prevalence [of sickle-cell anemia] among Caucasians is only 1 in about 58,000, compared to 1 in 500 African Americans and 1 in 1,000 to 1,400 Latino Americans.** "

How Prevalent Are Genetic Disorders?

The prevalence of genetic disorders varies widely because there are so many different types. For instance, according to the American Heart Association, as many as 1.3 million people in the United States suffer from congenital heart defects, although the actual number is likely much higher because individuals often do not know they have heart problems until symptoms appear. Breast cancer is the most common type of cancer among women in the United States. The National Cancer Institute estimates that more than 2 million American women suffer from breast cancer, and about 1 in 10 cases are hereditary.

There are many other genetic disorders as well. One of the most common is Down syndrome, which occurs in between 1 in 800 and 1 in 1,000 births in the United States and is a leading cause of mental retardation. Much less common is fragile X syndrome, which affects about 1 in 2,000 males and 1 in 4,000 females. Children who suffer from fragile X have mental impairment that ranges from learning disabilities to mental retardation, as well as physical characteristics such as a long face and large ears. An extremely rare genetic disorder is phenylketonuria (PKU), which occurs in about 1 out of 10,000 to 25,000 people. PKU affects the way the body processes protein, and if not treated immediately after birth, it can lead to severe mental retardation. A genetic disorder that primarily affects minorities is sickle-cell anemia. Prevalence among Caucasians is only 1 in about 58,000, compared to 1 in 500 African Americans and 1 in 1,000 to 1,400 Latino Americans.

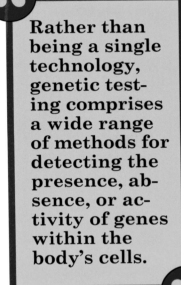

Rather than being a single technology, genetic testing comprises a wide range of methods for detecting the presence, absence, or activity of genes within the body's cells.

What Causes Genetic Disorders?

Genetic disorders occur as the result of defective genes that are passed to the baby from the mother, the father, or both. They are caused in whole or in part by mutations or variations in genes. Geneticists say that the gene variations involved in multifactorial inheritance disorders often occur in conjunction with environmental factors. Three examples of multifactorial inheritance disorders are congenital heart disease, breast cancer, and colon cancer. People who inherit the genes for these diseases have the potential to develop them, but may not necessarily do so. Their likelihood increases if they engage in unhealthy lifestyles such as smoking, excessive alcohol use, and being obese, or if they are exposed to viruses or toxic substances in the environment such as lead or mercury.

The Parental Age Factor

Studies have shown that the older a woman is when she becomes pregnant, the greater her chances of having a baby with certain genetic disorders. The March of Dimes states that pregnant women aged 25 have a 1 in 1,250 chance of having a baby with Down syndrome, while at age 49 the likelihood spikes to 1 in 10. According to a study that was published in April 2007, parental age also plays a role in the development of autism. The researchers found that the incidence of autism in children born to women younger than 20 years old was 1 in 251 births, compared to 1 in 123 for those born to mothers older than 40.

Even more significant was the connection between autism and advanced age in fathers. Those younger than 20 had a 1 in 387 chance of having a child with autism, and the odds jumped to 1 in 116 for fathers older than 40.

Diagnosis of Genetic Disorders

When symptoms are evident at birth, genetic disorders can usually be diagnosed by physical examinations and X-rays, as well as blood tests.

> " The fear of potentially developing cancer resulted in 11 members of a family opting for radical surgery: having their stomachs removed. "

One example is achondroplasia (a form of dwarfism), a genetic disorder that affects bone growth. The disorder is frequently obvious right away because babies are born with features such as a larger-than-normal head, a prominent forehead, and a nose that is flat at the bridge. The physical characteristics of Down syndrome are also usually evident at birth, including a slightly flattened face, eyes that slant upward, short toes with excessive space between the large and second toes, and single, deep creases across both palms. All newborns, even those who appear normal and healthy, are given routine screenings within a few days of birth. These screenings (the number of tests required varies from state to state) can identify potentially life-threatening genetic disorders that are not necessarily obvious, such as sickle-cell anemia, PKU, and galactosemia,

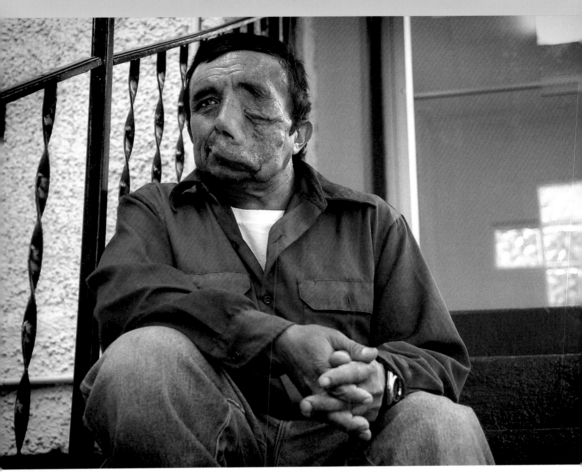

Manuel Raya, pictured a few months before undergoing reconstructive surgery, was born with neurofibromatosis, a single-gene genetic disorder that causes tumors to grow on the nerves and produces skin abnormalities and bone deformities. Raya's condition is more extreme than most others who have this disease.

a disease in which the body is unable to properly process a sugar known as galactose.

Some genetic disorders are not obvious at the time of birth and are not diagnosed until much later in life. For example, breast or colon cancer cannot usually be diagnosed until symptoms first begin to appear. Breast cancer may be detected at an early stage through a routine mammogram or later with biopsies, ultrasounds, and/or other types of screenings. Colon cancer may be detected through biopsies or computed tomography (CT) scans, which are X-ray tests that produce detailed cross-sectional images of the body.

Genetic Testing

Genetic testing has vastly improved over the years and now allows numerous genetic disorders to be diagnosed and treated, as the National Human Genome Research Institute explains:

> Genetic testing is available during pregnancy, and for diagnosis and treatment of infants, children and adults. . . . Gene tests look for signs of a disease or disorder in DNA taken from a person's blood, body fluids or tissues. The tests can look for large changes, such as a gene that has a section missing or added, or small changes, such as a missing, added, or altered chemical base within the DNA strand. Other important changes can be genes with too many copies, genes that are too active, genes that are turned off, or those that are lost entirely.[4]

Rather than being a single technology, genetic testing comprises a wide range of methods for detecting the presence, absence, or activity of genes within the body's cells. One type is prenatal testing, which can screen for genetic disorders such as Down syndrome in the fetus. If such a disorder is suspected, it can be confirmed or ruled out with diagnostic testing. Predictive testing shows if someone has a higher chance of getting a disease before symptoms appear, and presymptomatic testing is used to detect whether family members are at risk for a certain genetic condition. Carrier testing can tell individuals if they are carriers of a gene alteration for inherited disorders such as cystic fibrosis and Tay-Sachs.

How Should Genetic Test Results Be Used?

Although genetic tests have been shown to detect genetic disorders and, in the process, save lives, they are often a topic of heated debate. One source of controversy relates to people being tested to determine their likelihood for developing a disease such as Huntington's for which there is no treatment or cure. Genetics specialist Judy Garber urges caution in seeking such tests, as she explains: "You want to be sure you are ready to deal with the answer to the test. What if you find something? Have you considered what that will mean for you?"[5] Garber and other like-minded individuals say that discovering that such a devastating disease could strike at any time can make people fearful, anxious, and depressed decades before any symptoms are apparent.

Those who learn that they may be at risk of developing certain types of diseases that *can* be treated may, out of fear, opt to have radical operations. For example, women who find that they have inherited the BRCA1 or BRCA2 gene, which are associated with breast and ovarian cancer, often opt to have their breasts and/or ovaries removed as a precautionary measure. This was confirmed in a study published in March 2009, during which researchers at the University of Texas M.D. Anderson Cancer Center in Houston interviewed women who were tested for the gene mutation. Of those who tested positive, 81 percent underwent mastectomies— even though there was no certainty that they would actually develop cancer.

> According to the National Cancer Institute, the overall 5-year breast cancer survival rate in women is 87 percent, an increase of 15 percent since the 1970s.

The fear of potentially developing cancer resulted in 11 members of a family opting for radical surgery: having their stomachs removed. The cousins had all tested positive for a mutated gene known as CDH1 that causes an extremely rare, hereditary form of stomach cancer that had already claimed the lives of their grandmother and 6 of her children. The remaining family members who tested positive for the gene were told that they had a 70 percent chance of developing the cancer. Their only options were to wait and see or go ahead with the surgery, and they chose the latter. David Huntsman, the physician from British Columbia who discovered the genetic mutation in the family, explains their decision: "Rather than live in fear, they tackled their genetic destiny head-on."[6]

Treating Genetic Disorders

For some genetic disorders, such as color blindness and Huntington's disease, there are currently no treatments. Although cystic fibrosis is usually fatal before sufferers reach the age of 30, the disease can be treated with therapy to control infections and maintain lung function. Many people who suffer from multiple sclerosis can take medications that prevent further lesions from growing in their brains, which can make a remarkable difference in their muscle control. If PKU is detected during newborn screening, the baby is put on a special formula (and later diet) that has been shown to prevent mental retardation. The same is true with hypothyroidism, or underactive thyroid gland, which can also lead to mental retardation. If hypothyroidism is detected during newborn screening, the baby can be treated with oral doses of thyroid hormone supplements that can help ensure normal development.

Unlike years ago, when a diagnosis of congenital heart disease or cancer was virtually a death sentence, many people who develop these diseases can now live long, healthy lives. Heart defects can often be successfully treated with surgery combined with changing to a healthier lifestyle and diet. Chemotherapy and/or radiation kill cancerous cells in the body and can dramatically improve a patient's life expectancy, as can surgery in which cancerous tissue is removed. According to the National Cancer Institute, the overall 5-year breast cancer survival rate in women is 87 percent, an increase of 15 percent since the 1970s.

Can Genetic Disorders Be Cured?

Although scientists have made much progress in learning about genetic disorders and have developed treatments that improve people's quality of life, most of these disorders remain incurable. For instance, there is no cure for fragile X syndrome or cystic fibrosis, and both are fatal. Down syndrome cannot be cured, nor can muscular dystrophy or Alzheimer's disease. Many types of cancer, however, can be successfully treated, and many patients go into full remission, meaning that cancerous cells never return. There is also great hope for those with sickle-cell anemia, many of whom can become symptom free after bone marrow transplantation.

Throughout the years medical science has come a long way toward improving and saving the lives of people who suffer from cancer, heart defects, multiple sclerosis, and many other genetic disorders. Researchers continue to explore the thousands of disorders in an effort to discover more about their causes, as well as to develop improved treatments and therapies. In the future their discoveries may lead to methods of preventing and curing genetic disorders—and if that happens, the suffering of people who have them will finally become a thing of the past.

What Are Genetic Disorders?

❝As we unlock the secrets of the human genome, we are learning that nearly all diseases have a genetic component.❞

—National Human Genome Research Institute, which supports the development of resources and technology that will accelerate genome research and its application to human health.

❝Over the past decade, scientists have discovered specific inherited factors, or genes, that can contribute to the development of some forms of breast, ovarian, colorectal, and other types of cancer.❞

—Memorial Sloan-Kettering Cancer Center, the world's oldest and largest private cancer center.

In 1934 the mother of two mentally retarded children paid a visit to Norwegian physician Asbjørn Følling. Although he knew there was little or nothing he would be able to do for them, Følling agreed to examine the children. After taking urine specimens, he analyzed the samples and found that the urine was lacking in protein and glucose. Further analysis showed that the urine contained a chemical known as phenylpyruvic acid, which Følling theorized could be responsible for the children's mental retardation. He became convinced that this was the case after he learned that urine samples of eight other mentally retarded people contained the same substance. Følling had discovered the genetic disorder known as phenylketonuria (PKU).

In the decades since Følling's discovery, scientists have identified thousands of other genetic disorders, which are conditions that result from abnormal, or mutated, genes. These mutations occur because cells constantly divide and make copies of their own DNA, and sometimes these copies are defective. The difference from the original DNA sequence is a mutation. There are two general categories of genetic disorders: single gene and multifactorial. Single-gene disorders are caused by one particular gene, while multifactorial disorders are the result of both genetic and environmental factors.

A Hereditary Blood Disease

Of all the cells in the body, red blood cells perform one of the most vital functions. They constantly travel through the bloodstream, carrying oxygen from the lungs to tissues and organs, and then removing carbon dioxide, or cellular waste material. Normally, these microscopic blood cells are disk shaped, so they can easily fit through narrow blood vessels in order to carry out their work. An article in *Science Daily* explains the challenge of this process and how the blood cells overcome it: "As they flow through the body, they often encounter blood vessels, such as those in the brain, with a diameter of only about two microns. Each time the cells reach such a vessel, they must stretch into a bullet-like shape to squeeze through and then return to their original disc shape upon exiting the vessel."[7]

> "In a person with the genetic disorder sickle-cell anemia, blood cells are not disk shaped, but rather are shaped like crescents."

In a person with the genetic disorder sickle-cell anemia, blood cells are not disk shaped, but rather are shaped like crescents. The irregular shape makes it difficult for cells to flow through blood vessels properly, which creates blockages in the vessels. This can lead to a condition known as anemia (low blood count) that causes an individual to feel lethargic and exhausted, and it can also result in severe infections. Another effect of this abnormal flow of red blood cells is chronic pain in many parts of the body, including the spine, bones, joints, and abdomen. According to the Mayo Clinic, these bouts of pain may last anywhere from a few hours to weeks at a time. Some people with sickle-cell anemia suffer from just a few such episodes a year, while others have them much more frequently.

People with sickle-cell anemia can also suffer from life-threatening problems. For instance, studies have shown children with the disease have a more than 200 times greater risk of suffering a stroke than children who are not affected by it. This was the case with 6-year-old Ashton Taylor, who had been diagnosed with sickle-cell anemia when she was a new-born. On June 1, 2006, Ashton complained to her mother of severe pains in her stomach, and she was admitted to the hospital the following day. On June 6 she was transferred to another medical facility, where she underwent blood transfusions. Shortly afterward she began to feel better and had enough energy to sit up in bed and draw pictures—but her physical improvement did not last. Two days later Ashton again complained of pain and feeling uncomfortably hot throughout the day. That evening she suffered a stroke and the following day she died.

> " A multifactorial disorder that is not obvious at the time of birth (and often takes many years before symptoms appear) is colon cancer, which is the fourth most common type of cancer in the United States. "

Multifactorial Disorders

Genetic disorders are hereditary, but for those in the multifactorial group, environmental factors can also contribute. One example is cleft lip and palate, which is a deformation in the upper lip, upper gum, and/or soft tissue in the back of the mouth (soft palate). According to scientist Ingrid Lobo, even if parents are unaffected by the disorder, they may still pass defective genes that are required for lip and palate formation along to a child. "Indeed," she writes, "there seems to be a genetic component to this defect, because the incidence of cleft lip and palate is higher in families with an affected child."[8] Lobo adds that cleft lip and palate is a multifactorial genetic disorder because environmental factors such as nutritional deficiencies and smoking during pregnancy have been associated with the disorder.

A multifactorial disorder that is not obvious at the time of birth (and often takes many years before symptoms appear) is colon cancer, which is the fourth most common type of cancer in the United States. According to internal medicine specialist Dennis Lee, approximately 130,000 men and women develop colon cancer each year, and more than 50,000 die from it. He adds that the lifetime overall risk for people to develop colon cancer is approximately 6 percent, but for those who have a parent or sibling with the disease, the risk increases to 18 percent. In addition to genetic factors (mutated genes that can be inherited from one or both parents), environmental factors such as exposure to radiation, chemicals, and/or viruses may also act as triggers for development of colon cancer.

Prolific Tumors

One example of a single-gene disorder is neurofibromatosis (NF), a disease that affects the nervous system. The result is that benign (noncancerous) tumors, known as neurofibromas, grow along nerve tissue as well as on or under the skin. According to the National Institute for Neurological Disorders and Stroke (NINDS), the tumors begin in the cells that make up the myelin sheath, a thin membrane that surrounds and protects nerve fibers. Once tumors appear they often begin to spread into adjacent areas. A person who suffers from NF often has wartlike tumors growing on many different parts of the body, including arms, legs, hands, feet, face, and neck. In many cases these tumors are annoying to the individual but not serious, although there is a possibility that they may become cancerous.

Scientists have classified neurofibromatosis into 2 types: NF1 and NF2. The most common is NF1, which occurs in an estimated 1 in 4,000 births in the United States. Symptoms of NF1, particularly tumors or discolorations on the skin (known as café-au-lait spots), are often evident during infancy and almost always by the time a child has reached the age of 10. The NINDS states that with most cases of NF1, symptoms are mild and patients live normal and productive lives. NF2 is much rarer, occurring in about 1 in 50,000 births, and is far more serious. People who have NF2 often have tumors on both sides of the eighth cranial nerve, the nerve that is responsible for transmitting information from the inner ear to the brain. As the tumors grow, they cause pressure damage to the cranial nerve as well as to neighboring nerves. NF2 is not usually diagnosed until the teenage years or later, and side effects include hearing loss, tinnitus (continuous ringing in the ears), headaches, facial pain or numbness, and problems with balance. In some cases of NF2, tumors that develop on the brain and spinal cord can be life threatening.

The Most Common Fatal Genetic Disease

Of the numerous genetic disorders, cystic fibrosis is one of the most frightening for those who suffer from it because it often claims lives at a young age. According to the National Human Genome Institute, cystic fibrosis is the most common fatal genetic disease in the United States. People with the disease have an improper salt balance in their cells, which leads to the formation of a thick, sticky mucus that clogs the lungs, leads to infection, and blocks the pancreas from working properly. As a result, most people who suffer from cystic fibrosis do not live past their twenties or thirties. One person who died from the disease at age 25 was Frankie Abernathy, a cast member of the MTV reality program *Real World San Diego*. Even though Abernathy suffered from cystic fibrosis, her death was unexpected, as her mother explains: "It was very sudden. . . . She was doing fine, and we really don't know very much yet. It still was kind of a shock, and it just wasn't how we figured things would go. It seems like her little body just gave out."[9]

Kate Smith, who was diagnosed with cystic fibrosis at the age of 5, knows what it is like to live with the fear of an early death. But Smith, who lives in the United Kingdom, has far surpassed her doctors' predictions that she would not live to see her twenties. Now 30 years old, she says that in the back of her mind, "there is always a number—the average life expectancy for someone with my disease. That number is 31." Since people with cystic fibrosis have frequent infections, scarring develops in the lungs, and those who have it, as Smith explains, "will either slowly suffocate—leaving their lungs unable to supply enough oxygen to the body—or their immune system loses the battle against infections." Smith says that when she has developed infections, this has brought on "appalling pains in my chest and either side of my spine."[10]

> **According to the National Human Genome Institute, cystic fibrosis is the most common fatal genetic disease in the United States.**

In order to keep her disease under control, Smith must take as many as 50 prescription pills per day, regularly use inhalers to help her breathing, and get intravenous antibiotics through a permanent tube in her arm if she develops a serious infection. Despite the odds against her, Smith remains physically active and lives life to its fullest. "I'm having a big fundraising party on my 31st birthday, the day I overtake my life expectancy," she writes. "I have no idea how long I will live. . . . I know that when I die, it will be peaceful. In the meantime, I'm as busy as ever, making the most of my time."[11]

A Devastating Skin Disorder

In July 2007 a baby girl was born to parents in Saudi Arabia, and a videotape shot in the hospital was widely circulated on the Internet. Cruelly nicknamed "snake baby," the newborn's mouth was wide open, her eyes were bulged, and her face and body were horribly disfigured by a rare genetic disorder known as Harlequin ichthyosis (also called Harlequin disease). Babies who suffer from the disorder have diamond-shaped scales on their bodies separated by deep cracks, and their skin grows as fast overnight as a normal human's does in a week. This results in a thickened, scaly layer of skin that encases the body and greatly restricts movement of the arms and legs. Whatever movement is possible is dangerous for the baby because the cracks deepen and let in deadly bacteria that can cause severe infections. As a result, most babies who are born with Harlequin ichthyosis die shortly after birth. The baby girl who was born in Saudi Arabia only lived for a few hours.

> " Cruelly nicknamed "snake baby," the newborn's mouth was wide open, her eyes were bulged, and her face and body were horribly disfigured by a rare genetic disorder known as Harlequin ichthyosis. "

Ellie Luther, a little girl from Newcastle, England, is one child who has managed to beat the odds against her. Ellie was born with Harlequin ichthyosis and now, at nine years old, she is one of the few children in the world who have survived the disorder. She has no eyelids or ears and endures great pain because her excess layers of skin must be scrubbed off every three hours, and then greasy cream and bandages applied in order to protect her from infection. Ellie's father, Will Luther, says that when his daughter was born, treatment had to start immediately, as he explains: "As soon as she was born we had to start creaming her and cutting away at her skin, I just couldn't bring myself to do it because she was so small and fragile."[12] Yet in spite of her condition, and the pain that she endures every day, Ellie is a happy, well-adjusted little girl. She smiles often, is enthusiastic about life, and enjoys going to school and playing with her dolls.

A Complex Medical Issue

There is no one definition for the term *genetic disorders* because there is a multitude of different types. Each has its own individual symptoms, health risks, and frequency, but the one thing they all share in common is that genetics are involved. As research has progressed throughout the years, scientists have continued to identify additional types of genetic disorders as well as gain a great deal of knowledge about them. Yet many aspects of genetic disorders are still mysterious and unknown. Hopefully future research will reveal their many secrets.

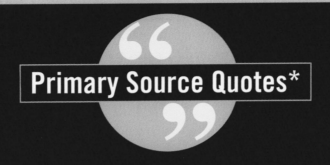

Primary Source Quotes*

What Are Genetic Disorders?

❝Down syndrome is the most commonly occurring genetic condition.❞

—National Down Syndrome Society, "About Down Syndrome: Myths and Truths," 2009. www.ndss.org.

The National Down Syndrome Society's mission is to be the national advocate for the value, acceptance, and inclusion of people with Down syndrome.

❝Sickle cell anemia is an inherited blood disorder that mostly affects people of African ancestry, but also occurs in other ethnic groups, including people who are of Mediterranean and Middle Eastern descent.❞

—James Fahner, "Sickle Cell Anemia," Kids Health, June 2007. http://kidshealth.org.

Fahner is the division chief of the Pediatric Hematology/Oncology Department at DeVos Children's Hospital in Grand Rapids, Michigan.

* Editor's Note: While the definition of a primary source can be narrowly or broadly defined, for the purposes of Compact Research, a primary source consists of: 1) results of original research presented by an organization or researcher; 2) eyewitness accounts of events, personal experience, or work experience; 3) first-person editorials offering pundits' opinions; 4) government officials presenting political plans and/or policies; 5) representatives of organizations presenting testimony or policy.

" Most genetic disorders are multifactorial inheritance disorders. Heart disease and most cancers are examples of these disorders. "

—University of California–San Francisco Memory and Aging Center, "Genetics," 2008. http://memory.ucsf.edu.

The Memory and Aging Center provides quality care for people with cognitive problems, conducts research on the causes and cures for degenerative brain diseases, and educates health professionals, patients, and their families.

" Achondroplasia is a genetic disorder of bone growth that is evident at birth. . . . Its depiction in ancient Egyptian art makes it one of the oldest recorded birth defects. "

—March of Dimes, "Achondroplasia," September 2008. www.marchofdimes.com.

The March of Dimes is dedicated to improving the health of babies by preventing birth defects, premature birth, and infant mortality.

" Red-green color deficiency is the most common form of color blindness; a less common form is blue-yellow color deficiency. "

—Gretchyn Bailey, "Color Blindness," All About Vision, June 2007. www.allaboutvision.com.

Bailey is a former optometric technician who has contributed to *Review of Optometry, Journal of the American Optometric Association,* and other vision-related publications.

66 Of the other major cardiovascular risk factors, choles-terol abnormalities . . . diabetes, high blood pressure (hypertension) and obesity are among those with the strongest hereditary components. **99**

—Amy Tucker, "Spotlight On: Hereditary Heart Disease," Club Red, 2009. www.clubreduva.com.

Tucker is a cardiologist at the University of Virginia Health System.

66 A tendency toward heart disease or fatty buildups in arteries seems to be hereditary. That means children of parents with heart and blood vessel diseases may be more likely to develop them. **99**

—American Heart Association, "Heredity as a Risk Factor," 2009. www.americanheart.org.

The American Heart Association's mission is to build healthier lives that are free of cardiovascular diseases and stroke.

66 Problems with chromosomes that result in genetic syndromes, such as Down syndrome, often result in a higher incidence of infant heart malformations. **99**

—St. Louis Children's Hospital, "Factors Contributing to Congenital Heart Disease," 2009. www.stlouischildrens.org.

The St. Louis Children's Hospital is known as one of the premier children's hospitals in the United States.

❝Hereditary diffuse gastric cancer is an inherited condition that greatly increases the risk of developing
stomach cancer.**❞**

> —American Cancer Society, "What Are the Risk Factors for Stomach Cancer?" May 14, 2009. www.cancer.org.

The American Cancer Society is dedicated to preventing cancer, saving lives, and
diminishing suffering from cancer through research, education, advocacy, and
service.

Facts and Illustrations

What Are Genetic Disorders?

- According to the National Institute of Neurological Disorders and Stroke, at least **500,000 people** in the United States suffer from Parkinson's disease.

- The National Fragile X Foundation states that about **1 in 3,600 to 4,000 males** throughout the world, and **1 in 4,000 to 6,000 females**, are born with the full gene mutation for fragile X.

- According to the National Institutes of Health, Down syndrome is the most common genetic cause of mild to moderate mental retardation and occurs in **1 out of 800 live births**.

- The American Heart Association estimates that between **650,000 and 1.3 million people** in the United States suffer from congenital heart defects.

- According to the National Institutes of Health, red-green color vision defects affect about **8 percent** of men and **0.5 percent** of women with northern European ancestry, while blue-yellow color vision defects affect males and females equally.

- The National Heart, Lung, and Blood Institute states that cystic fibrosis is one of the most common inherited diseases, affecting about **30,000 people** in the United States.

- According to the Memorial Sloan-Kettering Cancer Center, about **5 to 10 percent** of all female breast and ovarian cancer cases are hereditary.

Common Versus Rare Genetic Disorders

There are thousands of different genetic disorders and some are much rarer than others. This graph shows the prevalence among newborns of six genetic disorders. Congenital heart defects are the most common genetic disorder, affecting 1 out of 25 newborns.

Genetic disorder prevalence—1 out of . . .

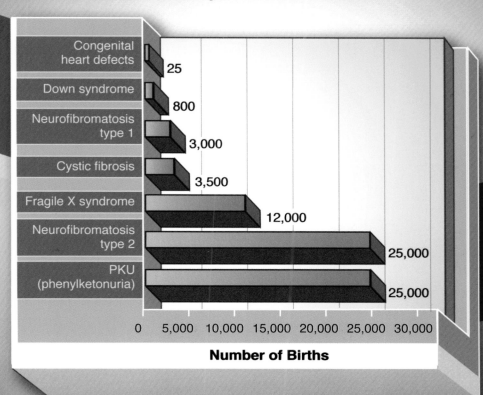

Number of Births

Sickle-Cell Anemia

Sickle-cell anemia is a potentially fatal disease that results in red blood cells being crescent-shaped (sickled) instead of the normal disk shape. This causes the cells to form clumps and get stuck in blood vessels, rather than being able to move freely throughout the body delivering oxygen from the lungs to organs and tissues. These blockages can lead to severe pain, serious infections, and organ damage. This illustration shows the difference between normal red blood cells and those that are produced in someone with sickle-cell anemia.

Cross-section of RBC

Normal red blood cells

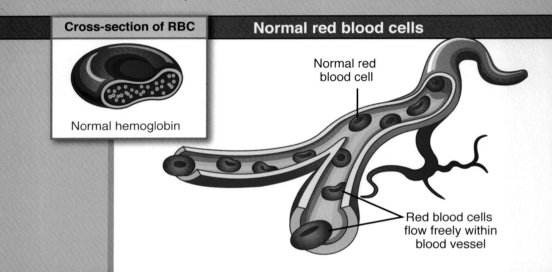

Normal hemoglobin

Normal red blood cell

Red blood cells flow freely within blood vessel

Cross-section of sickle cell

Abnormal, sickled, red blood cells (sickle cells)

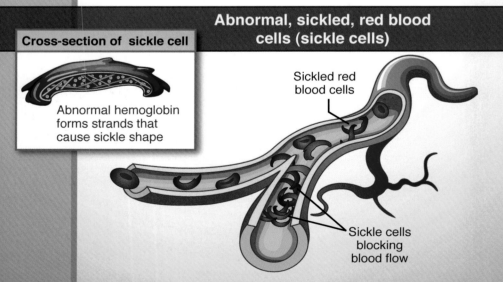

Abnormal hemoglobin forms strands that cause sickle shape

Sickled red blood cells

Sickle cells blocking blood flow

Source: National Heart, Lung, and Blood Institute, "Sickle Cell Anemia," August 2008. www.nhlbi.nih.gov.

- Although Alzheimer's disease generally affects those who are over the age of 65, people sometimes develop **"early onset" Alzheimer's** in their thirties and forties, and these individuals have a mutation in 1 of 3 different inherited genes.

- According to the National Human Genome Research Institute, when both parents are carriers of the defective gene that causes Tay-Sachs disease, each child has a **25 percent** chance of having Tay-Sachs and a **50 percent** chance of being a carrier.

Hereditary Forms of Cancer

The National Cancer Institute states that many types of cancer are hereditary, including cancer of the breast, colon and/or rectum, pancreas, kidney, bladder, and prostate. This graph shows the estimated number of cases diagnosed in the United States during 2009, as well as the estimated number of deaths.

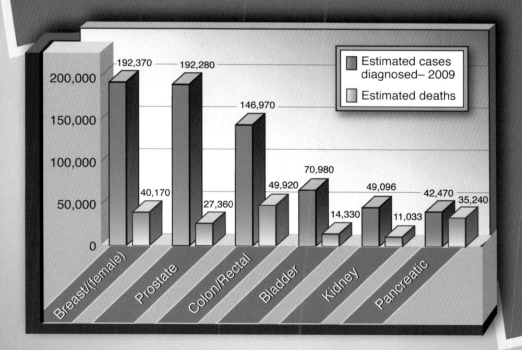

- Huntington's disease affects about **30,000 people** in the United States. According to the National Human Genome Research Institute, an additional **35,000 people** exhibit some symptoms, and **75,000 people** carry the abnormal gene that will cause them to develop the disease.

- If a parent has one of the two mutated genes that cause colon cancer, his or her children have a **50 percent** risk of inheriting the gene.

What Causes Genetic Disorders?

66 In hereditary genetic disorders, a mutated gene (one with changes in the DNA) that causes disease is passed down through generations of a family. 99

—University of California–San Francisco Memory and Aging Center, which provides quality care for people with cognitive problems, conducts research on the causes and cures for brain diseases, and educates health professionals, patients, and their families.

66 Every cell in the body has chromosomes containing genes that determine a person's unique characteristics. One missing or faulty gene can cause a birth defect. 99

—Linda Nicholson, a certified genetics counselor from Glenside, Pennsylvania.

K ris Bakowski was 46 years old when she received some devastating news—a diagnosis of early onset Alzheimer's disease. This is an extremely rare type, one that is hereditary and strikes people as young as 35, as opposed to late onset Alzheimer's, which usually does not become apparent until after age 65. According to the National Institutes of Health, the early onset type (also known as familial Alzheimer's disease) is caused by 1 of 3 gene mutations on chromosomes 1, 14, and 21. If someone inherits even 1 of these mutated genes from a parent, the person is almost certain to develop the disease, and his or her children also have a 50-50 chance of developing it. Both of Bakowski's parents died when they were in their early sixties, and she has no way of knowing which of them passed the mutated gene along to her. She suspects, though, that her grandfather may have suffered from Alzheimer's disease.

Soon after she was diagnosed, Bakowski wrote about the effects of the disease in her blog: "I've certainly been in a funk lately. I have no desire to do anything . . . don't want to go to work, don't want to get out of bed, don't want to socialize, nothing. I'm sure it is depression but I hate it when this happens." Bakowski also shared a frightening experience she had as a result of her memory loss, which is the hallmark of Alzheimer's disease. "The other night I was on my way home from work and couldn't make it home. I got disoriented and had to call my husband to come rescue me. I hate to be dependent on people. And knowing that dependency looms large in my future is depressing."[13]

Today, Bakowski is 53 years old, and memory loss and confusion have become an unfortunate fact of life for her. She tries to maintain a positive attitude, however, and works as an advocate for people who suffer from Alzheimer's. "Hopefully," she writes, "my perspective can and will help others."[14]

Genetics and Environment

Environmental factors have been linked to many hereditary diseases and disorders, and this can increase someone's risk of developing them. For instance, just because breast or colon cancer, heart disease, or arthritis runs in an individual's family, it does not necessarily mean that he or she will develop one of those diseases. Environmental factors such as smoking, excessive use of alcohol, lack of exercise, and/or an unhealthy diet have been shown to play a role.

Another example is diabetes, a disease in which the body does not produce or properly use insulin. With lower-than-normal levels of insulin, the body is not able to convert sugar, starches, and other food into the energy that it needs. Nearly 18 million people in the United States have been diagnosed with diabetes, although the American Diabetes Association (ADA) estimates that another 5.7 million have the disease and are not aware of it. The exact cause of diabetes is a mystery to scientists, but it is believed that both genetics and environmental factors are involved. The ADA explains: "Genes alone are not enough. One proof of this is identical twins. Identical twins have identical genes. Yet when one twin has type 1 diabetes, the other gets the disease at most only half the time. When one twin has type 2 diabetes, the other's risk is at most 3 in 4."[15]

A number of environmental factors have been linked to diabetes. For instance, type 1, which develops during childhood and is thought to involve genes inherited from both parents, develops more often in the winter than the summer and is more common in cold climates than in areas with warmer temperatures. This has long been puzzling to scientists, but in February 2008 a team of researchers from the University of Chicago announced that they may have solved the mystery. After studying genetic variations in more than 1,000 people from 54 different populations, the researchers found a strong connection between genes that helped early humans adapt to cold climates and disorders such as heart disease, high cholesterol, and diabetes.

Type 2 diabetes, which is far more prevalent than type 1, is also hereditary and is even more influenced by environmental factors. For instance, the disease is only common among people living in Western countries who typically eat diets that are high in fat and low in carbohydrates and fiber. The ADA states that people who live in areas without Westernized lifestyles almost never develop type 2 diabetes, no matter how strong their genetic risk may be. A close connection between high-fat diets and diabetes is obesity. According to the National Institute of Diabetes and Digestive and Kidney Diseases, more than 85 percent of people who have type 2 diabetes are overweight.

> " The exact cause of diabetes is a mystery to scientists, but it is believed that both genetics and environmental factors are involved. "

Metabolic Genetic Disorders

An estimated 1 in 4,000 people inherit metabolic disorders, which comprise a wide variety of medical problems that interfere with the body's metabolism, or the complex process by which the body turns food into energy. Researchers say that these disorders are caused by mutated genes that are usually passed to a child from both parents. The National Institutes of Health explains how metabolism normally works: "Metabolism is the process your body uses to get or make energy from the food you eat. Food is made up of proteins, carbohydrates and fats. Chemicals in your digestive system break the food parts down into sugars and acids, your body's fuel. Your body can use this fuel right away, or it can store the energy in your body tissues, such as your liver, muscles and body fat."[16]

When someone has a metabolic disorder, the normal chemical reactions in the body are disrupted.

One example of an inherited metabolic disorder is maple syrup urine disease (MSUD), which is so named because the urine of infants who have it smells sweet, much like maple syrup. Although scientists are not certain why, MSUD occurs much more frequently among members of the Old Order Mennonites, a group of Christian denominations that live simply, often without modern technology. It affects an estimated 1 in 185,000 infants worldwide, but among the Mennonite population the estimated prevalence is 1 in 380. Babies who are born with MSUD lack the ability to metabolize certain amino acids properly, and this can be life threatening. If infants with the most severe forms of MSUD are not diagnosed and treated soon after birth, they are at risk of having convulsions, lapsing into a coma, and dying.

> "One example of an inherited metabolic disorder is maple syrup urine disease (MSUD), which is so named because the urine of infants who have it smells sweet, much like maple syrup."

Another serious hereditary metabolic disorder caused by mutated genes is Tay-Sachs. Babies who have Tay-Sachs lack a vital enzyme known as hexosaminidase A (hex A), which is necessary for the body to break down a fatty waste substance that is found in brain cells. Without hex A, toxins build up in the brain cells and eventually destroy them. Tay-Sachs is extremely rare among the general population, and its prevalence is scattered among various groups, as the National Institutes of Health explains:

> The genetic mutations that cause this disease are more common in people of Ashkenazi (eastern and central European) Jewish heritage than in those with other backgrounds. The mutations responsible for this disease are also more common in certain French-Canadian communities of Quebec, the Old Order Amish community in Pennsylvania, and the Cajun population of Louisiana.[17]

The most common type of Tay-Sachs disease is apparent in babies, who typically appear normal until the age of three to six months and then begin to exhibit symptoms. At that point their development slows, their muscles become weaker, and they lose motor skills such as sitting, crawling, and rolling over. As the disease progresses, affected infants become blind, deaf, mentally retarded, and nonresponsive, and they usually do not live past the age of five.

One child who was born with Tay-Sachs—and has so far beaten the odds against her—is Krystie Anna Karl-Steiger, a 3-year-old girl from Rancho Mirage, California. Like most babies with Tay-Sachs, Krystie seemed perfectly fine for the first 6 months. Then, after the family returned home from a vacation in Cape Cod, her parents began to notice that she was not developing like other children her age. They explain: "We started to become very concerned when at 8 months she still could not sit or hold her own bottle. We then took her to a gym for babies aged 3 to 11 months and noticed that the 6 month olds seemed more alert and advanced than Krystie was at 9 months. She still could not sit, or clap and made no attempt at crawling." After going through a series of tests, Krystie was diagnosed with Tay-Sachs disease. She underwent a blood transfusion procedure in 2007, and although her body is now producing the missing enzyme, no one knows whether the enzyme will get to her brain in time to slow down or stop the disease from progressing. "Only time will tell,"[18] her parents write. Yet they have far more hope now than they did when their daughter was first diagnosed.

> As [Tay-Sachs] disease progresses, affected infants become blind, deaf, mentally retarded, and nonresponsive, and they usually do not live past the age of five.

Passing Genes from Parents to Children

One reason that genetic disorders are so complex is that they are caused by thousands of different gene mutations. Also, the faulty genes may be passed along to children from both parents or just one parent. Color blindness, for example, is caused by mutations only on the X chromosome, which girls inherit from their mothers or fathers and boys inherit only from their mothers. So, even if a father is color-blind, he can only pass the disorder on to his daughters and not to his sons. The same is true of fragile X syndrome, which is caused by a mutation on the FMR1 gene that is located on the X chromosome. According to the March of Dimes, fragile X affects about 1 in 4,000 males and 1 in 8,000 females across all racial and ethnic groups. Because men cannot pass along the X gene to their sons, boys who have fragile X syndrome always inherit the disorder from their mothers, whereas girls can inherit it from either parent.

The Strongest Toddler in the World?

Because so many genetic disorders have devastating consequences, it is difficult to imagine one that is not associated with any medical problems. But that is the case with a hereditary condition known as myostatin-related muscle hypertrophy. It is caused by mutations in a gene responsible for making myostatin, a protein that prevents muscles from growing too large. People with myostatin-related muscle hypertrophy have low body fat and develop muscle mass that is up to twice as much as normal. As a result, they often possess amazing strength. The disorder is extremely rare, and while its exact prevalence is not known, only a few people in the world are believed to have it.

> **People with myostatin-related muscle hypertrophy have low body fat and develop muscle mass that is up to twice as much as normal. As a result, they often possess amazing strength.**

Three-year-old Liam Hoekstra is one of the few. The western Michigan toddler appears to be perfectly normal—he looks and behaves just like most children his age. But that is where the similarity ends, as journalist Jeff Alexander writes: "When Liam picks up two five-pound dumbbells and waves them around like stuffed animals, or does rapid-fire sit-ups, it becomes abundantly clear that he has an extraordinary gift. In short, he's strong as a bull." Alexander adds that Liam has 40 percent more muscle mass than other children his age. "He is terrifically strong, quick as a rabbit, has the metabolism of a gerbil and almost no body fat."[19] Because Liam is adopted, his parents do not know the origin of the mutated gene that caused his condition. They believe, however, that he may have inherited myostatin-related muscle hypertrophy from his biological father, who was said to possess phenomenal strength.

Causes Galore

The question, "What causes genetic disorders?" is often answered with the cryptic response: "That depends." From the brain-wasting Alzheimer's disease to the muscle-pumping myostatin-related muscle hypertrophy, thousands of such disorders have been identified by scientists. The only thing they have in common is genetics—all are passed to children through the genes of one or both parents. In many cases, environmental factors such as unhealthy lifestyles contribute to the development of genetic disorders. As scientists continue to study the various types, they will undoubtedly uncover many of the secrets that still abound, including the multitude of genetic and environmental factors that contribute to their development.

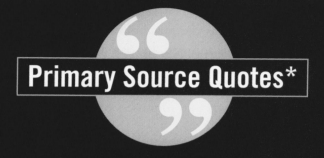

What Causes Genetic Disorders?

66 **Multifactorial inheritance means that 'many factors' are involved. The factors that produce the trait or condition are usually both genetic and environmental, involving a combination of genes from both parents.** 99

—University of Virginia Health System, "Overview of Mood Disorders," January 24, 2008. www.healthsystem.virginia.edu.

The University of Virginia Health System's mission is to provide excellence and innovation in patient care, the training of health professionals, and the creation and sharing of health-related knowledge.

66 **In some cases, genetic defects may contribute to brain malformations and 'miswiring' of nerve cell connections in the brain, resulting in cerebral palsy.** 99

—March of Dimes, "Cerebral Palsy," December 2007. www.marchofdimes.com.

The March of Dimes is dedicated to improving the health of babies by preventing birth defects, premature birth, and infant mortality.

* Editor's Note: While the definition of a primary source can be narrowly or broadly defined, for the purposes of Compact Research, a primary source consists of: 1) results of original research presented by an organization or researcher; 2) eyewitness accounts of events, personal experience, or work experience; 3) first-person editorials offering pundits' opinions; 4) government officials presenting political plans and/or policies; 5) representatives of organizations presenting testimony or policy.

66 Fragile X syndrome is transmitted from parent to child through the genetic information (DNA) that is present in the sperm and eggs.99

—National Fragile X Foundation, "How Is Fragile X Syndrome Inherited?" 2008. www.fragilex.org.

The National Fragile X Foundation provides educational and emotional support for those who have fragile X syndrome, as well as promotes public awareness of the disorder and advance research toward improved treatments and an eventual cure.

66 Color-blind fathers pass the gene to their daughters only, who will have normal color vision unless their mother also carries the color-deficient gene.99

—Gretchyn Bailey, "Color Blindness," All About Vision, June 2007. www.allaboutvision.com.

Bailey is a former optometric technician who has contributed to *Review of Optometry, Journal of the American Optometric Association,* and other vision-related publications.

66 Scientists have identified several genetic mutations associated with [Parkinson's disease], and many more genes have been tentatively linked to the disorder.99

—National Institute of Neurological Disorders and Stroke, "Parkinson's Disease: Hope Through Research," May 27, 2009. www.ninds.nih.gov.

An agency of the National Institutes of Health, the National Institute of Neurological Disorders and Stroke's mission is to reduce the burden of neurological disease.

66 A single gene disorder, also referred to as a monogenic disorder, is an inherited genetic disease that may develop due to a mutation, or defect, in just one gene. **99**

—Natural Standard Monograph, "Single Gene Disorders," 2008. www.naturalstandard.com.

Natural Standard Monograph's mission is to provide objective, reliable information that helps clinicians, patients, and health-care institutions to make more informed and safer therapeutic decisions.

....

66 Sometimes when an egg and sperm unite, the new cell gets too many or too few chromosomes. Most children born with Down syndrome, which is associated with mental retardation, have an extra chromosome number 21. **99**

—Louis E. Bartoshesky, "The Basics on Genes and Genetic Disorders," Teens Health, April 2009. http://kidshealth.org.

Bartoshesky is a pediatrician and medical geneticist.

....

What Causes Genetic Disorders?

- According to the National Institute of Mental Health, studies examining the occurrence of autism spectrum disorders (ASD) in siblings and family members suggest that **90 percent** of ASD involves genetic components.

- The Environmental Protection Agency states that along with genetics, environmental factors such as toxins, infectious agents, or diet may contribute to someone developing **type 1 diabetes**.

- The National Institutes of Health states that in more than **90 percent** of cases, Down syndrome is caused by the presence of an extra chromosome 21 in all the individual's cells.

- According to the March of Dimes, pregnant women aged 25 have a **1 in 1,250** chance of having a baby with Down syndrome, while at age 49 the likelihood increases to **1 in 10**.

- The National Heart, Lung, and Blood Institute states that **cystic fibrosis** is caused by a defect in the CFTR gene, which makes a protein that controls the movement of salt and water in and out of the body's cells.

- According to the National Human Genome Research Institute, Huntington's disease is caused by a **single abnormal gene** on chromosome 4.

- The National Heart, Lung, and Blood Institute states that when people have **sickle-cell anemia**, they have inherited two copies of the sickle-cell gene, one from each parent.

- Colon cancer is a **multifactorial disorder**, and according to the National Institutes of Health, people who have high-fat, low-fiber diets are most likely to develop it.

Cystic Fibrosis Most Prevalent Among Caucasians

Cystic fibrosis is a genetic disorder that is caused by abnormalities in a gene known as CFTR. Although the disease affects males and females of all races, it is far more prevalent among Caucasians.

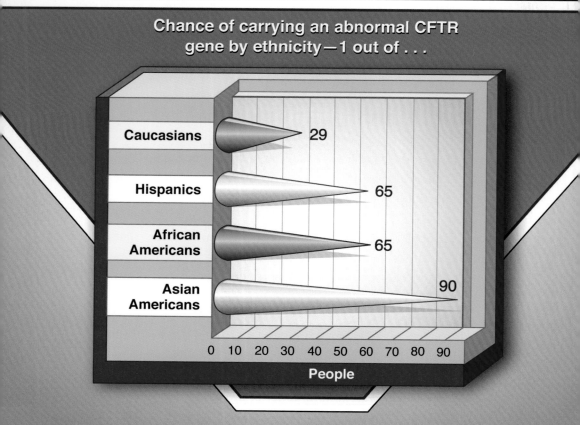

Chance of carrying an abnormal CFTR gene by ethnicity—1 out of . . .

- Caucasians: 29
- Hispanics: 65
- African Americans: 65
- Asian Americans: 90

People

Source: March of Dimes, "Cystic Fibrosis," March 2009. www.marchofdimes.com.

Single-Gene Disorders

All genetic disorders are linked to genes in some way but the particular gene mutations that cause them may vary widely. Single-gene disorders are usually caused by one particular gene, but that gene may have several different mutations. Those differences can determine the nature and severity of the disorder. This table shows five single-gene disorders, the genes that cause them, and the functions of those genes.

Condition	Gene That Causes Disorder	Gene Function
Cystic fibrosis	CFTR	Provides instructions for making a channel that transports chloride ions into and out of cells, which helps control the movement of water in tissues and is necessary for the production of thin, freely flowing mucus.
Duchenne muscular dystrophy	DMD	Provides instructions for making a protein called dystrophin, which plays a crucial role in muscle function.
Huntington's disease	HTT	Provides instructions for making a protein called "huntingtin" that plays a role in ensuring healthy neurons (brain cells).
Sickle-cell anemia (sickle-cell disease)	HBB	Provides instructions for making hemoglobin, a protein in red blood cells that allows them to carry oxygen from the lungs to tissues and organs in the body.
Tay-Sachs disease	HEXA	Provides instructions for making enzymes that are critical for proper function of the brain and spinal cord.

Multifactorial Disorders

Although many genetic disorders are caused by mutations in a single gene, the majority are multifactorial disorders, meaning they result from a combination of genetic and environmental factors. The faulty genes are inherited, which makes someone at increased risk for developing a disorder. Unless certain environmental factors are present, however, he or she may never develop the condition at all. Some of the most common multifactorial disorders are heart disease, diabetes, certain types of cancer, and rheumatoid arthritis.

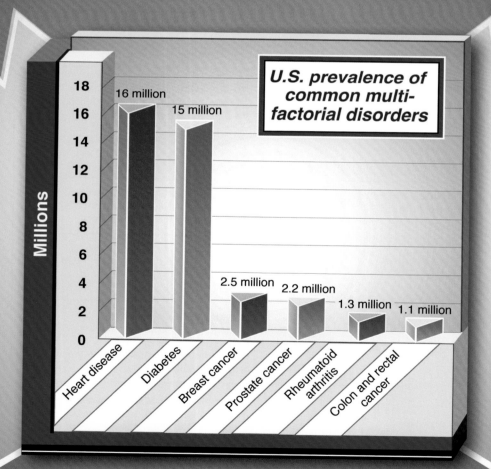

U.S. prevalence of common multi-factorial disorders

- Heart disease: 16 million
- Diabetes: 15 million
- Breast cancer: 2.5 million
- Prostate cancer: 2.2 million
- Rheumatoid arthritis: 1.3 million
- Colon and rectal cancer: 1.1 million

Sources: American Cancer Society, "Cancer Prevalence: How Many People Have Cancer?" October 30, 2008. www.cancer.org; American Heart Association, "Heart Disease and Stroke Statistics," 2008. www.americanheart.org; Carol Galbreath, "Arthritis Burden Soaring, Experts Say," Arthritis Foundation, January 2, 2008. www.arthritis.org.

- Fragile X syndrome is caused by a **mutated gene** on the X chromosome, one of the two sex chromosomes.

- Normally, females inherit one X chromosome from their mother and one X chromosome from their father, but those who have **Turner syndrome**, which involves physical problems ranging from major heart defects to minor cosmetic issues, are missing one of their X chromosomes.

- The most common type of a potentially fatal hereditary disorder known as **severe combined immunodeficiency** is caused by a mutation in the SCIDX1 gene located on the X chromosome.

- According to the March of Dimes, in about **50 percent** of cases, the abnormal gene that causes neurofibromatosis is inherited from one parent who has the disorder.

How Should Genetic Test Results Be Used?

❝ The way I think of it, genetic tests pull back the corner of a heavy curtain. The results give you a hint, a clue as to where you should consider paying more attention. ❞

—Hsien-Hsien Lei, a genetics information specialist at DNA Direct.

❝ Genetic diagnosis and intervention hold great promise. However, we need to consider carefully the power conferred on us by knowing our genetic identity and being able to alter it. ❞

—Margaret R. McLean, director of biotechnology and health-care ethics at the Markkula Center for Applied Ethics.

In 2007, after losing her mother-in-law to ovarian cancer, Susan Gilmore began thinking about the prevalence of cancer in her own family. Her maternal grandmother had died while in her early thirties, and no one seemed to know why. Gilmore also recalled that an aunt had died of ovarian cancer, and she became frightened about her own risk for developing the disease. Genetic testing had shown that her mother-in-law had one of the mutations in the BRCA1 gene, which has been linked to breast and ovarian cancer. Because of her own family history, Gilmore decided to get tested herself—and the news was not at all what she had hoped for. She tested positive for a genetic mutation that could potentially lead to cancer, but in her case it was quite possible that she would never develop it. Still, she was afraid to take even a small risk, and she decided to have her healthy ovaries surgically removed.

Beth Peshkin, Gilmore's genetic counselor, says that she can relate to the woman's state of mind and that for her, the surgery may have been

50

the best answer. But she also worries about the fact that more and more healthy people are getting genetic tests that often yield inconclusive results, which can cause them to make radical life decisions based solely on fear. When asked whether people like Gilmore are better off having genetic tests, Peshkin expresses doubt: "I don't know. In some ways probably yes, in some ways probably no. But this is what it is to live with uncertainty. And some people have a harder time living with uncertainty than others."[20]

Genetic Testing and Incurable Disease

Many people who are concerned about a family history of genetic disorders opt to have testing because they believe it will give them peace of mind—for them, just knowing is better than waiting to see what happens. Those for whom heart disease, diabetes, or cancer runs in the family could adopt healthier lifestyles to help reduce their risk, such as quitting smoking and/or eating more nutritious diets. Women who learn that they carry the mutated gene for breast cancer could also take precautions, like becoming diligent about performing breast self-examinations, getting more frequent mammograms, and watching closely for warning signs such as lumps in the breast. But what about someone who is potentially at risk for developing a disease such as Huntington's or early onset Alzheimer's? Both are devastating brain-wasting diseases for which there is no cure, and both are fatal. According to some genetics specialists, knowing about the risk ahead of time accomplishes nothing because nothing can be done to stop the disease. Because of that, people who may not become sick for many years may be consumed by stress and fear.

> Many people who are concerned about a family history of genetic disorders opt to have testing because they believe it will give them peace of mind—for them, just knowing is better than waiting to see what happens.

Katharine Moser is someone who chose to be tested for Huntington's. Her family has a strong history of the disease, and she hoped that she did not carry the mutated gene. But if she tested positive, she believed this would help her make decisions about how best to live her life. The test was positive—she learned that she does, in fact, carry the Huntington's gene. As a result of the test, Moser decided that marriage was no longer an option for her and she would never have children. Although she did not regret being tested, she felt a great deal of despair over knowing that she would eventually develop Huntington's disease. As Amy Harmon writes in the *New York Times*: "At night, crying herself to sleep in the dark of her lavender bedroom, she would go over and over it. She was the same, but she was also different. And there was nothing she could do."[21]

The Prenatal Testing Debate

One of the most controversial types of genetic testing is prenatal screening, which the American College of Obstetricians and Gynecologists recommends for *all* pregnant women, regardless of age. Previously the tests used to diagnose genetic disorders in a fetus, such as amniocentesis and chorionic villus sampling, involved inserting a needle into the uterus. Because those tests are invasive, a woman who undergoes either of them risks having a miscarriage. But now tests exist that are noninvasive. They simply involve testing a sample of the pregnant woman's blood, and they have been shown to be as accurate as the invasive tests.

> Studies have shown that among women carrying fetuses who test positive for Down syndrome, an estimated 90 percent choose to have an abortion.

Women who undergo prenatal screening are able to find out ahead of time whether their babies are likely to be born with one or more genetic disorders. If the test results are positive, the woman has the option of continuing with the pregnancy or terminating it—and that is an issue rife with controversy because such a large number of these pregnancies are aborted. For instance, studies have shown that among women carrying fetuses who test positive for Down syndrome, an estimated 90 percent choose to have an abortion. People who are against abortion, even if there is a strong possibility that the fetus has a genetic disorder, say that such a trend is akin to mass murder.

Yet those who disagree say that it is the mother's choice whether she wants to have the child or not. Rahul K. Parikh, a physician from San Francisco, insists that no one has the right to tell a woman that she must raise a child with special needs. He explains: "Rabid anti-choice activists have called that trend eugenics via medicine. But try telling that to a mother who is told early on in her pregnancy that she will be raising a child who will have a host of medical and developmental problems, requiring intense medical and social attention for the rest of his or her life. It can be tragic and nearly impossible news to bear."[22]

> After embryonic testing is performed, embryos that are found to be free of genetic mutations can be implanted in the mother's womb to initiate a pregnancy.

Another aspect of the prenatal testing controversy is that the test results are not always correct. This was the experience of Becky and Kriss Kramer, a couple from the United Kingdom. When Becky was pregnant, an MRI scan showed that the fetus had a rare brain disorder that could lead to deafness and blindness. She and her husband were told that their son would likely only survive a few hours after he was born. The doctor recommended abortion, but the Kramers refused—and on October 1, 2007, Becky gave birth to a perfectly healthy baby boy. "I feel incredibly guilty thinking that I could have killed him," she says, "and then I find myself wondering how many other babies are killed who would have turned out to be completely healthy."[23]

Testing Embryos

Parents who conceive children through in vitro fertilization, in which an egg is manually fertilized by sperm in a laboratory dish, can have their embryos tested for genetic disorders in a process known as preimplantation genetic diagnosis. One technique, called a "genetic MoT," was announced by researchers in the United Kingdom in October 2008. According to an article in the British newspaper the *Guardian*, the test is capable of detecting almost any known genetic disease in a two-day-old embryo, from

Huntington's disease and cystic fibrosis to cancer and muscular dystrophy, as well as thousands of others. It could also be used to assess the risk of developing heart disease, cancer, and/or Alzheimer's disease later in life.

After embryonic testing is performed, embryos that are found to be free of genetic mutations can be implanted in the mother's womb to initiate a pregnancy. This is an issue that is fraught with ethical concerns because the leftover "defective" embryos are almost certain to be destroyed by the fertility clinic at the parents' request. Josephine Quintavalle, who heads the group Comment on Reproductive Ethics, says that she is disturbed by this type of screening because carriers of the gene do not always develop the disease, and even if they do, the disease is not necessarily fatal. She explains: "The message we are sending is: 'Better off dead than carrying (a gene linked to) breast cancer.' We have gone very much down the proverbial slippery slope."[24]

Genetic Testing in Children

There is disagreement over whether children should be subjected to genetic testing. People who are in favor of it argue that it is best to have the knowledge because it is more harmful to be uncertain about whether children may eventually develop genetic disorders. Those who oppose such procedures argue that children could be harmed psychologically by test results and could suffer from fear and anxiety if they learn that they could develop serious diseases in the future. This, opponents say, could lead to adverse family and social relationships, interference with normal development of self-esteem, and feelings of failure in the child.

According to BreastCancer.org, even if there is a strong family history of breast cancer, most experts advise against children under the age of 18 undergoing testing for genetic mutations that cause breast cancer. As its Web site explains:

> No safe, effective therapies currently exist to help prevent breast cancer in children so young. Furthermore, children are not yet old enough to decide for themselves whether they want information about their lifetime cancer risks. It is also possible that by the time today's children reach adulthood, scientists will have discovered a new treatment to correct abnormal breast cancer genes before cancer has a chance to develop.[25]

One type of genetic test that was announced in 2009 has sparked a fierce debate about genetic testing in children. A Colorado company, Atlas Sports Genetics, offers to analyze DNA samples of children as young as one year old to help predict whether they will have superior athletic ability when they are older. The procedure is simple: Parents swab inside a child's cheek and along the gums to obtain samples of DNA. Then they seal the swab into a sterile bag and return it to the company for analysis. Atlas Sports Genetics tests the sample to evaluate a gene known as ACTN3, which has been shown to be linked to athletic prowess. Those who are against such tests argue that positive results could motivate parents to push their children too hard to excel in sports. As health and fitness journalist Peta Bee explains: "That does not sit easily with my parental instinct, which is to expose my three-year-old to the diversities of life, including sport, in the hope that he will choose to pursue hobbies that he is good at, but mostly that he enjoys. Could I be trusted to do that if I was armed with results from a gene test that may suggest that he is steered towards a specific activity? I am not so sure."[26]

> A Colorado company, Atlas Sports Genetics, offers to analyze DNA samples of children as young as one year old to help predict whether they will have superior athletic ability when they are older.

Can Genetic Testing Lead to Discrimination?

Until recently, one risk of genetic testing was that those who tested positive for the likelihood of a genetic disorder could possibly be fired from their jobs if employers found out about the result. The same was true of health insurance companies: If they learned that a policyholder was at risk for developing a disease that could result in expensive medical procedures, the person could lose his or her coverage. This happened to Heidi Williams, a woman from Kentucky, whose son and daughter carry a mutated gene that can lead to liver failure and lung problems such as emphysema. They are not predisposed to illness because they each only carry one gene. In spite of that, however, when Williams tried to get health insurance, she was rejected by the insurer because she had been required to disclose the information about her children's genetic testing.

As of May 2008, with the passage of the Genetic Information Non-discrimination Act, such discrimination is no longer legal. Under this legislation, employers cannot discriminate against employees based on genetic testing, and insurance companies are prohibited from denying coverage, adjusting premiums, or exhibiting any form of discrimination based on genetic test results. One aspect of the law is that not only does it prevent employment or insurance discrimination based on genetic test information, it also prohibits companies from requesting or receiving it.

What Is the Answer?

There is no doubt that some genetic testing is beneficial. People can learn whether they have a higher-than-normal risk of developing treatable problems such as cancer and heart disease and can take steps to reduce their risk. But what is gained by determining that one is highly likely, or even certain, to develop incurable, untreatable diseases such as Huntington's? Or finding out that a child may potentially develop a serious disease decades later? Some believe that knowing ahead of time is better than living in a constant state of uncertainty. Others, however, are not so sure.

"A woman has the absolute right to choose to have an abortion, including the right to abort a fetus diagnosed with [a] physical handicap."

—Nicholas Provenzo, "The Fundamental Right to Abortion," Opposing Views, February 17, 2009. www.opposingviews.com.

Provenzo is chair of the Center for the Advancement of Capitalism.

"As science extends our capabilities to detect more and more conditions in the womb, as it inevitably will, I can't help asking if perhaps we should pause to ask if knowledge is always power. Should we have the right to determine who does and who doesn't get to inhabit the world?"

—Rebecca Atkinson, "My Baby, Right or Wrong," *Guardian*, March 10, 2008. www.guardian.co.uk.

Atkinson is a woman from the United Kingdom who suffers from a rare genetic disorder known as Usher syndrome.

* Editor's Note: While the definition of a primary source can be narrowly or broadly defined, for the purposes of Compact Research, a primary source consists of: 1) results of original research presented by an organization or researcher; 2) eyewitness accounts of events, personal experience, or work experience; 3) first-person editorials offering pundits' opinions; 4) government officials presenting political plans and/or policies; 5) representatives of organizations presenting testimony or policy.

Primary Source Quotes

"There is general agreement among the medical community that genetic testing holds great promise for diagnosis and treatment of many diseases, but determining who should get a genetics test, how to interpret results, and if it can accurately predict risk, is a big challenge facing clinicians today."

—American Academy of Physician Assistants, "Learning the Universe of Genetic Testing," *AAPA News,* November 30, 2008. www.cdc.gov.

The American Academy of Physician Assistants is a professional organization that represents physician assistants across medical and surgical specialties in all 50 states, the District of Columbia, Guam, the armed forces, and the federal services.

"I think genetics has a huge amount to offer in making really important real-time health-care decisions. I think increasingly we're going to see genetic testing as being really important in both prescribing decisions and in treatment decisions."

—Kathy Hudson, interviewed by Claudia Kalb, "Beware Genetic Snake Oil," *Newsweek,* April 3, 2008. www.newsweek.com.

Hudson is the founder and director of the Genetics and Public Policy Center at Johns Hopkins University.

"Knowing you'll develop a disease—or at least have that chance—could be devastating. If there's no cure or effective treatment for the condition, you may feel helpless in facing the years ahead."

—Emily Carlson, "Living with Huntington's," National Institute of General Medicine, *Findings,* September 2008. http://publications.nigms.nih.gov.

Carlson is a science writer for the National Institute of General Medicine.

❝There are some within the Huntington's community who believe that it is more courageous to test.❞

—LaVonne Veatch Goodman, "To Test or Not to Test: The Elephant in the Picture Window," Huntington's Disease Drug Works, December 28, 2007. http://hddrugworks.org.

Goodman is a physician and the founder of Huntington's Disease Drug Works, an organization that provides information about treatment options, drug development, and human clinical trials to people who have Huntington's disease.

❝Many in the medical establishment feel that uncertainties surrounding test interpretation, the current lack of available medical options for these diseases, the tests' potential for provoking anxiety, and risks for discrimination and social stigmatization could outweigh the benefits of testing.❞

—Human Genome Project, "Gene Testing," September 19, 2008. www.ornl.gov.

The Human Genome Project is a genetic research agency of the U.S. Department of Energy's Office of Science.

❝Genetic testing for potentially lethal disorders is an area fraught with ethical, legal, and social concerns.❞

—Karen Norrgard, "Ethics of Genetic Testing: Medical Insurance and Genetic Consideration," *Nature Education,* 2008. www.nature.com.

Norrgard is a scientist with Commonwealth Biologies.

66 Remember that individual genes are only part of the puzzle. A negative result can be reassuring, but it doesn't guarantee that you won't develop a disease. 99

—Mayo Clinic, "Genetic Testing: Insight from Mayo Clinic Specialists," January 31, 2008. www.mayoclinic.com.

The Mayo Clinic is a world-renowned medical practice that is dedicated to the diagnosis and treatment of virtually every type of complex illness.

66 It is critical for the public to realize that genetic testing is only one part of a complex process which has the potential for both positive and negative impact on health and well-being. 99

—American College of Medical Genetics, "ACMG Statement on Direct-to-Consumer Genetic Testing," April 7, 2008. www.acmg.net.

The American College of Medical Genetics provides education, resources, and a voice for the medical genetics profession.

Facts and Illustrations

How Should Genetic Test Results Be Used?

- **Genetic tests** are done on a small sample of blood, cells swabbed from the inside of the mouth, saliva, hair, skin, tumors, or the fluid that surrounds a fetus during pregnancy.

- According to the Genetics and Public Policy Center at Johns Hopkins University, there are **more than 1,500 different genetic tests**.

- The Human Genome Project says that in the United States, **no regulations** exist for evaluating the accuracy and reliability of genetic testing.

- The organization BreastCancer.org states that **removing the breasts and ovaries** to lower cancer risk **does not get rid of every breast- and ovary-related cell,** so a woman may still develop cancer in other tissues and organs.

- The American Association for Clinical Chemistry states that although genetic testing may detect a particular problem gene, it **cannot predict how severely the person carrying that gene will be affected.**

- According to the National Down Syndrome Society, certain diagnostic prenatal tests can predict whether a fetus has Down syndrome with nearly **100 percent accuracy.**

- Studies have shown that an estimated **90 percent** of women who learn that their baby will likely be born with Down syndrome choose to have an abortion.

Types of Genetic Tests

Doctors can predict or diagnose thousands of genetic diseases and disorders because of genetic testing capabilities. Such tests can save lives. A person who is genetically more likely to develop diabetes or heart disease may be able to make lifestyle changes to prevent onset of the disease. But genetic testing is also controversial. Prenatal testing can show the likelihood of a child being born with severe birth defects, which may lead to the mother having an abortion. Genetic testing can also tell whether a person is likely to develop a disease that has no cure, such as Huntington's disease. This knowledge may cause extreme fear and have a harmful effect on that person's life. This table shows the different types of genetic tests and their purposes.

Type of genetic test	Purpose
Newborn screening	Screens newborn babies for early detection of diseases such as sickle-cell anemia and PKU (phenylketonuria); if caught at this early stage, treatment may prevent the onset of symptoms or minimize the severity of the disease.
Carrier testing	Can help couples learn if they carry the genes for conditions such as cystic fibrosis, sickle-cell anemia, and Tay-Sachs disease, which could be passed along to their offspring.
Prenatal diagnostic testing	Detects changes in a fetus's genes or chromosomes that could potentially indicate the presence of a genetic disorder such as Down syndrome.
Diagnostic and/or prognostic testing	Used to confirm a diagnosis in someone who has symptoms of a disease or disorder, or to monitor the person's prognosis in response to treatment.
Predictive or pre-dispositional testing	Can identify the risk and/or probability of someone developing a disease before symptoms have appeared.

Source: Genetic Alliance, "Understanding Genetics NYMAC," June 2, 2009. www.resourcerepository.org.

- In June 2008 California's Department of Public Health found that **13 genetic testing companies** were in violation of state law by offering clinical laboratory tests directly to consumers without a physician's order.

- Under the **Genetic Information Nondiscrimination Act**, which was passed in May 2008, individuals are protected from discrimination initiated by an employer or health insurance company based on genetic test results.

How Americans View Genetic Testing

During a November to December 2008 survey by Virginia Commonwealth University, 1,005 adults nationwide were asked to share their perspective on genetic testing for various purposes. As this chart illustrates, an overwhelming majority felt either strongly positive or somewhat positive about such testing.

Genetic testing is being used to identify people at risk for diseases such as cancer, heart disease, Alzheimer's, and others. How much would you favor or oppose making genetic testing easily available to all who want it?

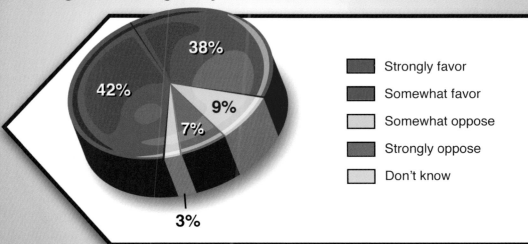

38%

42%

9%

7%

3%

- Strongly favor
- Somewhat favor
- Somewhat oppose
- Strongly oppose
- Don't know

Note: Total is slightly less than 100 percent due to rounding.

Source: Cary Funk, "VCU Life Sciences Survey 2008," Virginia Commonwealth University, December 2008. www.news.vcu.edu.

Perspectives on Abortions

In October 2007 Fox News conducted a survey of 900 registered voters in the United States to determine under what circumstances (if any) they would consider abortion to be acceptable. The participants' responses are indicated on this chart. Fifty-three percent of respondents said abortion should be allowed if the fetus has a fatal birth defect.

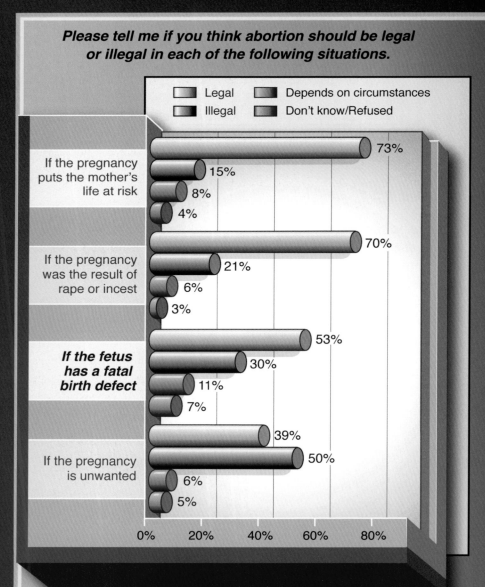

Please tell me if you think abortion should be legal or illegal in each of the following situations.

Legend:
- Legal
- Illegal
- Depends on circumstances
- Don't know/Refused

If the pregnancy puts the mother's life at risk
- 73%
- 15%
- 8%
- 4%

If the pregnancy was the result of rape or incest
- 70%
- 21%
- 6%
- 3%

If the fetus has a fatal birth defect
- 53%
- 30%
- 11%
- 7%

If the pregnancy is unwanted
- 39%
- 50%
- 6%
- 5%

Axis: 0% 20% 40% 60% 80%

Source: Fox News, "Opinion Dynamics Poll," October 26, 2007. www.foxnews.com.

Acceptability of Prenatal Genetic Testing

A study published in January 2009 by New York University's Langone Medical Center showed that people have a high desire for genetic testing under certain circumstances but do not feel favorably about it in other cases.

Percent of respondents who said prenatal genetic testing is acceptable for these traits and conditions:

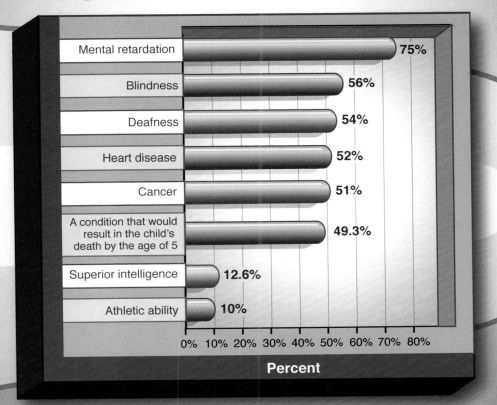

Source: New York University Langone Medical Center, "Consumers Desire More Genetic Testing, but Not Designer Babies," January 26, 2009. http://communications.med.nyu.edu.

- The American Cancer Society does not recommend widespread testing for the gene mutations that cause breast and ovarian cancer because these mutations are present in **less than 1 percent of the general population.**

Can Genetic Disorders Be Cured?

❝The NINDS supports and conducts research on genetic disorders . . . in an effort to find ways to prevent, treat, and ultimately cure these disorders.❞

—The National Institute of Neurological Disorders and Stroke (NINDS), whose mission is to reduce the burden of neurological disease.

❝With its potential to eliminate and prevent hereditary diseases such as cystic fibrosis and hemophilia and its use as a possible cure for heart disease, AIDS, and cancer, gene therapy is a potential medical miracle-worker.❞

—Linda Nicholson, a certified genetic counselor from Glenside, Pennsylvania.

In June 2008 researchers from the University of California–Los Angeles announced the results of a very promising study. It involved using mice that had been genetically engineered to have tuberous sclerosis complex (TSC), a genetic disorder that affects only 1 in 10,000 people. Although it is rare, the disorder is devastating because it causes tumors to form in many different organs, primarily the brain, eyes, heart, kidneys, and lungs. Like people who suffer from TSC, the mice had mental impairments, the source of which the researchers traced to abnormalities in the hippocampus, the part of the brain that plays a crucial role in memory. The mice were injected with rapamycin, a drug that is usually used to fight tissue rejection following organ transplants. Rapamycin was selected because it has been shown to target enzymes that are responsible for making proteins necessary for memory, and the same enzyme is also involved with TSC proteins. The researchers found that the drug reversed mental impairment in the mice, as UCLA's Dan Ehninger explains: "After only three days of treatment, the TSC mice learned as quickly as the healthy mice. The rapamycin corrected the biochemistry, reversed the learning deficits and restored normal hippocampal function, allowing the mice's brains to store memories properly."[27] The experiment netted a treatment rather than a cure, but the researchers believe that rapamycin could eventually offer hope to people with TSC by slowing or preventing the mental impairment that is associated with the disorder. Although this was just one of thousands of studies and it applied to a rare disorder, it illustrates how promising scientific research is in potentially leading to treatments and cures for many different genetic disorders.

The Promise of Stem Cells

Of all the research that is being done to further the understanding, treatment, and potential cures for genetic disorders, none has caused more excitement among scientists than studies with stem cells. Although there are trillions of cells in the human body, stem cells are the master cells that have the remarkable ability to create any cells in the body (known as differentiation). Embryonic stem cells come from three- to five-day-old embryos, and stem cells that come from adult tissue are known as adult stem cells. Researchers believe these unique cells hold tremendous promise for eventually curing a wide variety of genetic disorders, including Parkinson's disease, diabetes, cancer, and heart disease, as well as a genetic disorder of the nervous system known as Batten's disease, which begins in childhood and is fatal.

Stem cells have already been shown to cure the genetic disorder sickle-cell anemia in some people who have undergone treatments. One success story involves Joe Davis Jr., who was diagnosed at birth in 1999 and began to suffer serious symptoms when he was 8 months old. Joe often experienced high fevers and painful swelling in his hands and feet, and by the time he was 2 years old he had been hospitalized 20 times and had 3 blood transfusions. His parents checked all over the world to find a donor whose stem cells matched their son's, but they were not successful. Then, when his mother was pregnant with her second child, she had prenatal testing to see if the baby's stem cells matched Joe's, and she learned that they were an identical match. In 2002, after baby Isaac was born, stem cells were taken from his umbilical cord blood and transplanted into Joe—and a month later Joe was out of the hospital and healed. As of May 2008 Joe was 8 years old, healthy, and thriving, as his mother explains: "He's doing great and he's loving life. When he was little, the doctors told me he would have to take antibiotics every day for the rest of his life. Guess what? He's not taking anything. And I thank God for that."[28]

Saving a Little Boy's Life

Genetic diseases are usually considered incurable because even if they are successfully treated, the mutated genes remain in the body. But research is giving hope to many people who suffer from genetic disorders and have

> **Of all the research that is being done to further the understanding, treatment, and potential cures for genetic disorders, none has caused more excitement among scientists than studies with stem cells.**

not believed that a cure was possible. This is the case with Theresa Liao, who was prepared to do most anything to save her 18-month-old son, Nate. He had been born with a devastating genetic disorder known as epidermolysis bullosa (EB), which is considered to be incurable and is almost always fatal. The disorder occurs because the protein collagen VII, which acts as the glue that fuses the outermost and innermost layers of skin together, is lacking in the blood. In people with EB, huge, painful blisters form all over the body, and skin falls off at the slightest touch. "If you can imagine the worst blister you may get on your foot," Liao says, "multiply that by a thousand."[29] As with others who suffer from EB, Nate's blisters were inside his body as well as outside—so swallowing anything other than baby food caused abrasions to his esophagus. Without some sort of treatment, Liao knew that Nate would likely die before he reached young adulthood. She decided to let him undergo an experimental bone marrow transplant at the University of Minnesota, during which he would receive a transplant of healthy marrow from his older brother Julian. The goal of the procedure was for stem cells from the transplanted bone marrow to travel to Nate's skin and begin to make collagen. Although bone marrow transplants are often used to treat other genetic disorders, the procedure had never been used to treat EB, and there was a significant chance that it would not be successful—but it was.

Within weeks of having the bone marrow transplant, Nate was already showing noticeable improvement. Because cells were creating collagen in his bloodstream, he was no longer thin-skinned and pale, his face had begun to plump up, his skin had fewer blisters, and he was eating Oreo cookies. His physicians were optimistic that Nate had been cured and that he would continue to improve. "Maybe we can take one more disorder off the incurable list," says bone marrow specialist John Wagner. "It's not often that it feels like you hit a home run in medical research, but this one feels like it."[30] As of June 2009 Nate was still doing very well and continuing to improve.

Healing Bad Genes with Good Genes

Although gene therapy research is still in the experimental phase, it holds exciting promise for treating and potentially curing genetic diseases. According to the National Institutes of Health (NIH), researchers are testing several approaches with gene therapy. These include replacing a mutated gene with a healthy copy of the gene, inactivating a mutated gene that is functioning improperly, and introducing a new gene into the body to help fight a disease or disorder. "Gene therapy is designed to introduce genetic material into cells to compensate for abnormal genes or to make a beneficial protein," the NIH writes. "If a mutated gene causes a necessary protein to be faulty or missing, gene therapy may be able to introduce a normal copy of the gene to restore the function of the protein."[31] The NIH adds that in order for new genetic material to function, it must be delivered by a carrier called a vector, which is usually a virus that has been modified so it will not cause disease in humans. The vector carrying the healthy genes can either be injected into the patient's body or given intravenously.

> " **[Nate] had been born with a devastating genetic disorder known as epidermolysis bullosa (EB), which is considered to be incurable and is almost always fatal.** "

In March 2009 researchers from the United Kingdom announced that gene therapy studies with mice could potentially lead to a cure for many types of cancer. The scientists wrapped healthy "tumor-busting" genes in microscopic particles known as nanoparticles, and then inserted the packages into mice. Once inside, the genes began to stimulate production of a protein that destroyed cancer cells but did not harm healthy cells. Lead researcher Andreas Schatzlein explains: "Once inside the cell, the gene enclosed in the particle recognises the cancerous environment and switches on. The result is toxic, but only to the offending cells, leaving healthy tissue unaffected." This finding is promising because chemotherapy, the traditional cancer treatment, destroys all cells in the affected area, including those that are healthy, and it leads to side effects such as fatigue, nausea, and hair loss. "This is the first time that nanoparticles have been shown to target tumours in such a selective way," says Schatzlein, "and this is an exciting step forward in the field."[32] He adds that gene therapy may be available to start treating cancer patients in clinical trials in a couple of years.

> "Thus far, clinical trials with ataluren have shown great promise and have led to improvements among children and adults who suffer from Duchenne muscular dystrophy and cystic fibrosis."

Another successful experiment was announced in May 2009 by researchers from the University of Florida. A dog that was born with a genetic disorder known as glycogen storage disease type 1A (GSD1) appeared to have been cured by gene therapy. GSD1 is caused by a faulty enzyme that does not convert stored sugar (glycogen) to glucose, the type of sugar the body needs for energy. This prevents the body from getting needed energy and causes glycogen to build up in the liver. Although GSD1 is extremely rare, occurring in only about 1 in 50,000 births, it is dangerous because liver function is impaired. If it is not caught and treated immediately when symptoms first become apparent, children who have the disease risk seizures, permanent brain damage, and death.

The goal of the experiment was to use gene therapy to restore the faulty enzyme so the dog's body could use sugar properly. The dog was initially treated the day after she was born, and then she received a second treatment when she was five months old. At the time that the announcement was made, the dog was almost two years old, was eating regular dog food, and appeared to be perfectly healthy. Many in the scientific community are enthusiastic about the researchers' findings because of what they could mean for people who suffer from GSD1. Joseph Wolfsdorf, who is a pediatric specialist at Children's Hospital in Boston, shares his thoughts: "This is very exciting work and holds great promise for treatment of the disease in humans."[33]

A Pill to Cure Genetic Disorders?

All genetic disorders are in some way linked to genes. Many are caused by "nonsense mutations," meaning an alteration in the genetic code that prematurely halts the creation of essential proteins. Science writer Mark Henderson explains: "Genes are instruction manuals for cells to make proteins, but nonsense mutations in effect introduce a command halfway through that stops production. The kind of protein disrupted determines the nature of the disease."[34] One example is Duchenne muscular dystrophy, in which the protein necessary for normal muscle development is not created, which leads to the devastating muscle wasting that is characteristic of the disease.

> " Although gene therapy research is still in the experimental phase, it holds exciting promise for treating and potentially curing genetic diseases. "

Scientists have determined that a drug known as ataluren (formerly PTC124), which is taken orally, is effective at preventing nonsense mutations. The drug binds to the ribosome, part of a cell that translates genetic code into protein, which allows the ribosome to ignore the premature "stop signals" and continue forming functioning proteins. According to PTC Therapeutics, the developers of ataluren, the drug does not alter the patient's genetic code, nor does it introduce genetic material into the body. Thus far, clinical trials with ataluren have shown great promise and have led to improvements among children and adults who suffer from Duchenne muscular dystrophy and cystic fibrosis. Researchers are optimistic that the drug can eventually be used to treat other diseases caused by nonsense mutations, including beta-thalassemia, which is a blood disorder, and Hurler syndrome, which causes mental and physical impairment and is often fatal by the time a child is 10 years old.

What the Future Holds

Because there are thousands of different genetic disorders, it would be impossible for researchers to develop one miracle treatment that cures them all. Progress is being made, however, and there is more hope for people with many of these disorders than there ever was in the past. Stem cell treatments have been shown to cure sickle-cell anemia, and they have great potential for treating and curing a number of other diseases and disorders. Gene therapy and drug treatments also show immense promise for the future. Although research still has a long way to go before genetic disorders are wiped out, the number of people whose lives have been saved is tangible evidence of the progress scientists have made.

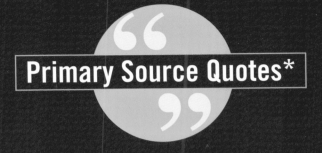

Primary Source Quotes*

Can Genetic Disorders Be Cured?

66 **Overcoming breast cancer is not easy, but advances in medical science help surgeons work miracles. Then it's down to the individual to decide what part their attitude can play in effecting a lasting cure.** 99

—Zola Jones, "Life in Remission: After Breast Cancer," Her Active Life, December 16, 2007. www.heractivelife.com.

Jones is a breast cancer survivor who writes motivational articles for other women suffering from the disease.

66 **Somewhere in the world, there's someone working hard to build a better mouse trap. In the meantime, a team . . . has figured out how to build a better 'knockout' mouse, a key research tool for exploring the genetic factors involved in health and disease.** 99

—National Human Genome Research Institute, "Making a Mightier Knockout Mouse," June 22, 2009. www.genome.gov.

The National Human Genome Research Institute supports the development of resources and technology that will accelerate genome research and its application to human health.

* Editor's Note: While the definition of a primary source can be narrowly or broadly defined, for the purposes of Compact Research, a primary source consists of: 1) results of original research presented by an organization or researcher; 2) eyewitness accounts of events, personal experience, or work experience; 3) first-person editorials offering pundits' opinions; 4) government officials presenting political plans and/or policies; 5) representatives of organizations presenting testimony or policy.

❝Luckily, we've gotten through . . . years of people saying, 'End-stage diabetic mice can't be cured.' So they're cured. Seven international labs all have very happy mice.❞

—Denise Faustman, interviewed by David Edelman, "Interview with Dr. Denise Faustman: Clinical Trial for a Type 1 Diabetes Cure," *Diabetes Daily,* September 2, 2008. www.diabetesdaily.com.

Faustman is a researcher whose laboratory was the first in the world to cure mice of a form of diabetes that closely resembles type 1 diabetes in humans.

❝[Embryonic stem cells] hold great promise for studying many genetic disorders, such as cystic fibrosis and Huntington's disease. The capacity to recreate these disease conditions in cells in the lab will help researchers look for new drugs.❞

—Peter Klatsky, "The Great Potential of Stem Cells," *Huffington Post,* March 9, 2009. www.huffingtonpost.com.

Klatsky is a physician who specializes in women's and reproductive health.

❝Sickle cell anemia affects millions of people worldwide. The disease has no widely available cure.❞

—National Institutes of Health, "What Is Sickle Cell Anemia?" August 2008. www.nhlbi.nih.gov.

The National Institutes of Health, which is part of the U.S. Department of Health and Human Services, is the primary federal agency for conducting and supporting medical research.

66 Researchers are making great strides in identifying the genes on Chromosome 21 that cause the characteristics of Down syndrome. Many feel strongly that it will be possible to improve, correct or prevent many of the problems associated with Down syndrome in the future. 99

—National Down Syndrome Society, "Down Syndrome Fact Sheet," 2009. www.ndss.org.

The National Down Syndrome Society's mission is to be the national advocate for the value, acceptance, and inclusion of people with Down syndrome.

66 At present, there is no cure for [Parkinson's disease], but a variety of medications provide dramatic relief from the symptoms. 99

—National Institute of Neurological Disorders and Stroke, "Parkinson's Disease: Hope Through Research," May 27, 2009. www.ninds.nih.gov.

An agency of the National Institutes of Health, the National Institute of Neurological Disorders and Stroke's mission is to reduce the burden of neurological disease.

66 Cystic fibrosis (CF) is an inherited disease that affects the lungs and digestive system. . . . Most affected individuals survive into their late 30s, though some die in childhood and others live to age 40 or beyond. There is currently no cure. 99

—March of Dimes, "Cystic Fibrosis," March 2009. www.marchofdimes.com.

The March of Dimes is dedicated to improving the health of babies by preventing birth defects, premature birth, and infant mortality.

Can Genetic Disorders Be Cured?

- About **90 percent** of patients survive colon cancer, which is caused by a combination of genetic and environmental factors, after treatment with chemotherapy, radiation, and/or surgery.

- A genetic disorder known as **phenylketonuria cannot be prevented or cured**, but children who are treated with a special diet that is low in the amino acid phenylalanine may recover completely.

- A study published in June 2008 showed that when the brains of rats genetically altered to have Parkinson's disease were **injected with stem cells** from the nose of Parkinson's patients, the creatures made a marked recovery.

- According to researchers from Children's Hospital of Pittsburgh and the Clinic for Special Children, 11 people suffering from a rare but deadly genetic disorder known as **maple syrup urine disease** were cured after receiving liver transplants.

- In May 2009 researchers from Spain announced that they had **successfully reprogrammed cells of patients** with the genetic disorder Fanconi anemia to become healthy cells, which could lead to human transplants that cure the disorder.

The Vast Potential of Stem Cells

Stem cells are the master cells from which all other cells in the body are made. Scientists are excited about stem cells because of their ability to be "reprogrammed" into other cells that could potentially cure a wide variety of diseases and disorders. In December 2007 scientists from the Massachusetts Institute of Technology (MIT) announced that they had cured sickle-cell anemia in mice by using stem cell treatment. This illustration shows the process used during such an experiment.

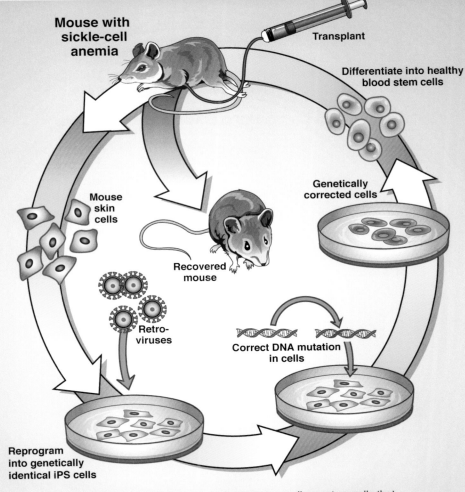

Mouse with sickle-cell anemia

Transplant

Differentiate into healthy blood stem cells

Genetically corrected cells

Mouse skin cells

Recovered mouse

Retro-viruses

Correct DNA mutation in cells

Reprogram into genetically identical iPS cells

Note: "iPS" indicates induces pluripotent stem cells, or stem cells that have been reprogrammed.

Source: Science Daily, "Adult Cells, Reprogrammed to Embryonic Stem Cell-Like State, Treat Sickle-Cell Anemia in Mice," December 7, 2007. www.sciencedaily.com.

- In December 2008 researchers announced that they had **successfully created the genetic disease spinal muscular atrophy in a laboratory dish** by using cells from a patient. This will allow them to watch the course of the disease as it progresses and potentially pave the way toward treatments or a cure.

Genetic Disorder Research Funding

Throughout the years, scientists have made great progress in identifying genetic disorders, studying them, and learning more about what causes them, and in the future this may lead to improved treatments and/or cures. The National Institutes of Health allocates billions of dollars each year to help make scientific research possible, although some diseases are given much higher priority than others, as this graph illustrates.

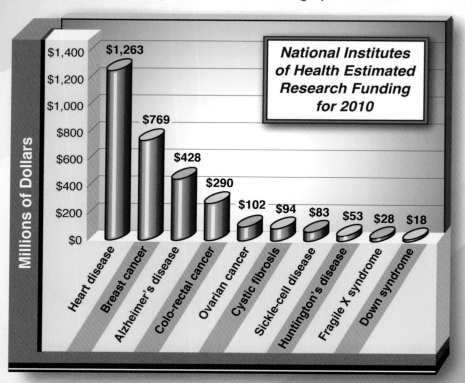

National Institutes of Health Estimated Research Funding for 2010

Millions of Dollars

Disease	Funding
Heart disease	$1,263
Breast cancer	$769
Alzheimer's disease	$428
Colo-rectal cancer	$290
Ovarian cancer	$102
Cystic fibrosis	$94
Sickle-cell disease	$83
Huntington's disease	$53
Fragile X syndrome	$28
Down syndrome	$18

Source: National Institutes of Health, "Estimates of Funding for Various Research, Condition, and Disease Categories (RCDC)," May 7, 2009. http://report.nih.gov.

The Lifesaving Potential of Bone Marrow Transplants

Inside bones is a soft, spongy material known as marrow, which contains stem cells that are capable of producing red blood cells, white blood cells, and platelets (cells that help blood to clot). With certain genetic disorders, a bone marrow transplant may replace diseased cells with healthy cells, and this can result in the disease being cured.

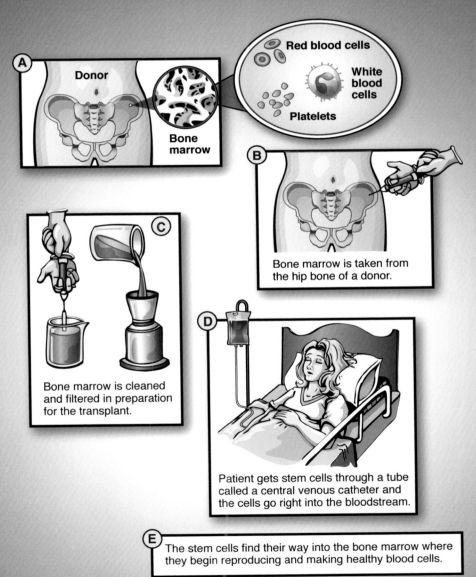

A — Donor / Bone marrow / Red blood cells / White blood cells / Platelets

B — Bone marrow is taken from the hip bone of a donor.

C — Bone marrow is cleaned and filtered in preparation for the transplant.

D — Patient gets stem cells through a tube called a central venous catheter and the cells go right into the bloodstream.

E — The stem cells find their way into the bone marrow where they begin reproducing and making healthy blood cells.

Source: National Institutes of Health, "Medical Encyclopedia: Bone Marrow Transplant," Medline Plus, October 30, 2008. www.nlm.nih.gov.

Key People and Advocacy Groups

Cure Tay-Sachs Foundation: A group that is dedicated to funding the research projects that provide hope for developing a treatment and/or cure for Tay-Sachs disease.

Cystic Fibrosis Foundation: An organization whose mission is to assure the development of the means to cure and control cystic fibrosis, as well as improve the quality of life for those with the disease.

Genetics Society of America: A group that seeks to foster a unified science of genetics and to maximize the science's intellectual and practical impact.

Robert A. Good: The physician who, in 1968, performed the first bone marrow transplant on an infant with a genetic immune deficiency disorder.

March of Dimes: An organization that is dedicated to improving the health of babies by preventing birth defects, premature births, and infant mortality.

Gregor Mendel: An Austrian scientist who published his laws of genetics in 1865 and eventually became known as the Father of Genetics.

National Down Syndrome Society: A group that focuses on being the national advocate for the value, acceptance, and inclusion of people with Down syndrome.

National Fragile X Foundation: An organization that enriches Fragile X victims' lives through educational and emotional support, promotes public and professional awareness, and advances research toward treatments and a cure for fragile X syndrome.

National Human Genome Research Institute: A group whose focus is on supporting the development of resources and technology that will accelerate genome research and its application to human health.

National Institute of Neurological Disorders and Stroke: An agency of the National Institutes of Health that is dedicated to reducing the burden of neurological disease throughout the world with research and education.

Sickle Cell Disease Association of America: An organization that works toward improving the quality of health, life, and services for anyone who is affected by sickle-cell disease and related conditions, while promoting the search for a cure.

James A. Thomson: The first scientist to isolate human embryonic stem cells in 1998, who in 2007 successfully reprogrammed normal human skin cells to have the same qualities as embryonic stem cells.

Chronology

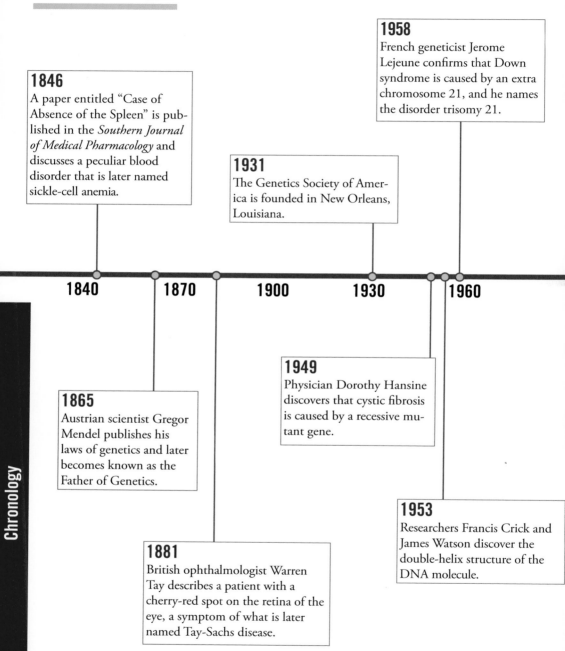

1958
French geneticist Jerome Lejeune confirms that Down syndrome is caused by an extra chromosome 21, and he names the disorder trisomy 21.

1846
A paper entitled "Case of Absence of the Spleen" is published in the *Southern Journal of Medical Pharmacology* and discusses a peculiar blood disorder that is later named sickle-cell anemia.

1931
The Genetics Society of America is founded in New Orleans, Louisiana.

1840   1870   1900   1930   1960

1949
Physician Dorothy Hansine discovers that cystic fibrosis is caused by a recessive mutant gene.

1865
Austrian scientist Gregor Mendel publishes his laws of genetics and later becomes known as the Father of Genetics.

1953
Researchers Francis Crick and James Watson discover the double-helix structure of the DNA molecule.

1881
British ophthalmologist Warren Tay describes a patient with a cherry-red spot on the retina of the eye, a symptom of what is later named Tay-Sachs disease.

Chronology

1968
Robert A. Good performs the first bone marrow transplant on an infant with a genetic immune deficiency disorder, and the patient is cured.

1997
The National Center for Human Genome Research is granted full institute status at the National Institutes of Health and becomes the National Human Genome Research Institute.

2009
Researchers from the Salk Institute for Biological Studies announce that after taking hair or skin cells from patients with the rare genetic disorder Fanconi anemia, they corrected the defective genes in a laboratory dish using gene therapy techniques.

1993
Scientists identify the DNA sequence and determine the precise nature of the gene mutation that is associated with Huntington's disease.

1970   1980   1990   2000   2010

1988
The first umbilical cord blood transplant cures a young boy from France who was born with the hereditary, potentially fatal blood disease Fanconi anemia.

2007
Two-year-old Nate Liao becomes the first person to be cured of the fatal genetic skin disorder epidermolysis bullosa after receiving a bone marrow transplant.

1995
A team of scientists reports that the anticancer drug hydroxyurea is the first treatment that can reduce the frequent, painful complications of sickle-cell disease.

2004
Researchers announce that they have found a fossil of a child that had a hereditary tooth disorder known as amelogenesis imperfecta; the fossil is estimated to be 1.5 million years old.

Related Organizations

American Cancer Society
250 Williams St., Suite 600
Atlanta, GA 30303
phone: (404) 320-3333; toll-free: (800) 227-2345
fax: (404) 982-3677
Web site: www.cancer.org

The American Cancer Society is dedicated to preventing cancer, saving lives, and diminishing suffering from cancer through research, education, advocacy, and service. Its Web site offers cancer facts and figures, stories of hope from cancer survivors, annual statistics, research information, and a search engine that links to numerous articles about hereditary forms of cancer.

American Heart Association (AHA)
National Center
7272 Greenville Ave.
Dallas, TX 75231
phone: (800) 242-8721
Web site: www.americanheart.org

The AHA's mission is to build healthier lives, free of cardiovascular diseases and stroke. Its Web site offers numerous publications about heart diseases and disorders, including a "Heart and Stroke Encyclopedia," fact sheets, statistics, and archived news releases.

Cure Tay-Sachs Foundation
12730 Triskett Rd.
Cleveland, OH 44111
phone: (216) 812-5855
fax: (216) 251-6728
e-mail: questions@curetay-sachs.org
Web site: www.curetay-sachs.org

The Cure Tay-Sachs Foundation is dedicated to funding the research projects that provide hope for developing a treatment and/or cure for Tay-

Sachs disease. Its Web site features real-life stories of people whose children were born with Tay-Sachs, as well as quarterly updates on research initiatives, a downloadable brochure, and statistics.

Cystic Fibrosis Foundation

Cystic Fibrosis Foundation (national headquarters)
6931 Arlington Rd.
Bethesda, MD 20814
phone: (301) 951-4422; toll-free: (800) 344-4823
e-mail: info@cff.org
Web site: www.cff.org

The Cystic Fibrosis Foundation's mission is to assure the development of the means to cure and control cystic fibrosis as well as improve the quality of life for those with the disease. Its Web site offers a wealth of information about cystic fibrosis, including the *Commitment* newsletter, research, news releases, frequently asked questions, and a "Living with Cystic Fibrosis" section.

Genetics Society of America

9650 Rockville Pike
Bethesda, MD 20814-3998
phone: (301) 634-7300; toll free: (866) 486-4363
fax: (301) 634-7079
Web site: www.genetics-gsa.org

The Genetics Society of America seeks to foster a unified science of genetics and to maximize its intellectual and practical impact. Its Web site offers news releases, highlights from the *Genetics* newsletter, and a search engine that links to genetic disorders articles.

March of Dimes

1275 Mamaroneck Ave.
White Plains, NY 10605
phone: (914) 997-4488
Web site: www.marchofdimes.com

The mission of the March of Dimes is to improve the health of babies by preventing birth defects, premature birth, and infant mortality. Its Web site offers medical reference fact sheets, research programs, statistics, and scientific publications and reports.

National Down Syndrome Society (NDSS)

666 Broadway, 8th Floor
New York, NY 10012
phone: (800) 221-4602
e-mail: info@ndss.org
Web site: www.ndss.org

The NDSS's mission is to be the national advocate for the value, acceptance, and inclusion of people with Down syndrome. Its Web site offers numerous fact sheets, position papers, questions and answers, and a "Myths and Truths" section.

National Fragile X Foundation

PO Box 37
Walnut Creek, CA 94597
phone: (925) 938-9300; toll-free: (800) 688-8765
fax: (925) 938-9315
Web site: www.fragilex.org

The National Fragile X Foundation enriches lives of fragile X victims through educational and emotional support, promotes public and professional awareness of the disorder, and advances research toward treatments and a cure for fragile X syndrome. Its Web site explains the family of fragile X conditions and provides information about causes, characteristics, and testing, as well as research and news releases.

National Human Genome Research Institute (NHGRI)

Building 31, Room 4B09
31 Center Dr., MSC 2152
9000 Rockville Pike
Bethesda, MD 20892-2152
phone: (301) 402-0911
fax: (301) 402-2218

Web site: www.genome.gov

The NHGRI, which is part of the National Institutes of Health, supports the development of resources and technology that will accelerate genome research and its application to human health. A wealth of information about genetic disorders can be found on its Web site, including research, articles, a multimedia presentation, fact sheets, ethical issues, and a search engine that produces nearly 800 articles.

National Institute for Neurological Disorders and Stroke (NINDS)

PO Box 5801
Bethesda, MD 20824
phone: (301) 496-5751; toll-free: (800) 352-9424
fax: (301) 402-2060
Web site: www.ninds.nih.gov

The NINDS, which is part of the National Institutes of Health, seeks to reduce the burden of neurological disease throughout the world with research and education. Its Web site features a comprehensive "Disorders A to Z" section, as well as a search engine that links to hundreds of articles related to genetic disorders and diseases.

National Institutes of Health (NIH)

9000 Rockville Pike
Bethesda, Maryland 20892
phone: (301) 496-4000
e-mail: nihinfo@od.nih.gov
Web site: www.nih.gov

The NIH is the United States' primary federal agency for conducting and supporting medical research. NIH scientists search for ways to improve human health as well as investigate the causes, treatments, and possible cures for diseases. Its Web site features news releases, archived issues of the NIH *News in Health* newsletter, information about research, and a search engine that produces nearly 16,000 articles when the term *genetic disorders* is entered.

Sickle Cell Disease Association of America (SCDAA)

231 E. Baltimore St., Suite 800
Baltimore, MD 21202
phone: (410) 528-1555; toll-free: (800) 421-8453
fax: (410) 528-1495
e-mail: scdaa@sicklecelldisease.org

The SCDAA's mission is to advocate for and enhance its members' ability to improve the quality of health, life, and services for anyone who is affected by sickle-cell disease and related conditions, while promoting the search for a cure. Its Web site features the *Sickle Cell News* newsletter, an "About Sickle Cell Disease" section, news articles, and research information.

For Further Research

Books

Clare Dunsford, *Spelling Love with an X: A Mother, a Son, and the Gene That Binds Them.* Boston: Beacon, 2007.

Michael J. Fox, *Always Looking Up: The Adventures of an Incurable Optimist.* New York: Hyperion, 2009.

Jeri Freedman, *Tay-Sachs Disease.* New York: Chelsea House, 2009.

Judy Monroe Peterson, *Sickle Cell Anemia.* New York: Rosen, 2008.

Kathryn Lynard Soper and Martha Sears, *Gifts: Mothers Reflect on How Children with Down Syndrome Enrich Their Lives.* Bethesda, MD: Woodbine House, 2007.

Alice Wexler, *The Woman Who Walked into the Sea: Huntington's and the Making of a Genetic Disorder.* New Haven, CT: Yale University Press, 2008.

James Wynbrandt and Mark D. Ludman, *The Encyclopedia of Genetic Disorders and Birth Defects.* New York: Facts On File, 2008.

Doris Teichler Zallen, *To Test or Not to Test: A Guide to Genetic Screening and Risk.* New Brunswick, NJ: Thorndike Press, 2009.

Periodicals

Laura Apel, "Cleft Lip and Cleft Palate—What to Know and Who Can Help," *Exceptional Parent*, August 2008.

Betsy Bates, "Silvery Hair Points to Deadly Genetic Syndromes," *Family Practice News*, January 1, 2009.

Maria Caroff, "Family Lives Life Fully in the Face of a Rare Genetic Disorder for All Three Children," *Exceptional Child*, May 2008.

Steve Maich, "Drugs Just for You: Genetic Testing Can Tell What Drugs Work Best, and Fastest, for Whom," *McLean's*, October 1, 2007.

Sheila Monaghan, "Know Your Roots (Genetic Disorders)," *Self*, February 2009.

Alan Mozes, "Obesity May Hide Fetal Abnormalities on Ultrasounds," *Consumer Health News*, April 22, 2009.

Regina Nuzzo, "Nabbing Suspicious SNPS: Scientists Search the Whole Genome for Clues to Common Diseases," *Science News*, June 21, 2008.

Tralee Pearce, "Risk of Birth Defects Linked to Month of Conception," *Globe & Mail* (Toronto), April 1, 2009.

Rachel Porter, "A Test Tube Timebomb?" *Daily Mail* (London), April 30, 2009.

Steven Reinberg, "Folic Acid Reduces Infant Heart Defects," *Consumer Health News*, May 12, 2009.

Andrea Stone, "The Day I Considered Abortion: Could I Trust God Despite My Baby's Potential Birth Defects?" *Today's Christian Woman*, March/April 2008.

M.D.W. Allan Walker and Courtney Humphries, "Starting the Good Life in the Womb," *Newsweek*, September 17, 2007.

Kirsten Weir, "Fortune Telling: Would You Take a Genetic Test to See What's in Store for Your Health?" *Current Science*, a *Weekly Reader* publication, February 27, 2009.

Internet Sources

Mary Hanan, "Meet the Boy Too Big for His Mom's SUV," ABC News, August 19, 2008. http://abcnews.go.com/Health/MedicalMysteries/story?id=5466774&page=1.

National Human Genome Research Institute, "Specific Genetic Disorders," April 14, 2009. www.genome.gov/10001204.

National Institutes of Health, "New Findings Raise Questions About Process Used to Identify Experimental Drug for Rare Genetic Diseases," February 2, 2009. www.nih.gov/news/health/feb2009/nhgri-02.htm.

Linda Nicholson, "Birth Defects," Kids Health, October 2007. http://kidshealth.org/parent/system/ill/birth_defects.html.

University of California–San Francisco, "Inherited Genetic Diseases Treatable with Stem Cells," April 1, 2008. http://fetus.ucsfmedicalcenter.org/stem_cells.

Source Notes

Overview

1. Quoted in Lisa Priest, "'I Know How I Am Going to Die,'" *Globe and Mail* (Toronto), April 3, 2009. www.theglobeandmail.com.
2. Quoted in Priest, "'I Know How I Am Going to Die.'"
3. Science Clarified, "Genetic Disorders," 2008. www.scienceclarified.com.
4. National Human Genome Research Institute, "Frequently Asked Questions About Genetic Testing," February 5, 2009. www.genome.gov.
5. Quoted in the Boston Channel, "Genetic Breast Cancer Testing Brings Controversy," October 9, 2007. www.thebostonchannel.com.
6. Quoted in Alicia Chang and Malcolm Ritter, "11 Cousins Have Their Stomachs Removed to Fight Risk of Cancer," *San Diego Union-Tribune*, June 19, 2006, p. A4.

What Are Genetic Disorders?

7. *Science Daily*, "How Blood Cells Change Shape," March 23, 2007. www.sciencedaily.com.
8. Ingrid Lobo, "Multifactorial Inheritance and Genetic Disease," *Nature Education*, 2008. www.nature.com.
9. Quoted in Chris Harris, "'Real World: San Diego' Alum Frankie Abernathy Dead At 25," MTV Networks, June 12, 2007. www.mtv.com.
10. Kate Smith, "Living with Cystic Fibrosis," *Daily Mail* (London), February 2008. www.dailymail.co.uk.
11. Smith, "Living with Cystic Fibrosis."
12. Quoted in Chris Robinson, "Little Ellie Really Is One in a Million," *JournalLive*, July 3, 2007. www.journallive.co.uk.

What Causes Genetic Disorders?

13. Kris Bakowski, "In a Funk," Dealing ith Alzheimer's Blog, January 29, 2004. http://creatingmemories.blogspot.com.
14. Kris Bakowski, "About Me," Dealing with Alzheimer's Blog, June 2009. http://creatingmemories.blogspot.com.
15. American Diabetes Association, "The Genetics of Diabetes." www.diabetes.org.
16. National Institutes of Health, "Metabolic Disorders," MedLine Plus, June 1, 2009. www.nlm.nih.gov.
17. Genetics Home Reference, "Tay-Sachs Disease," National Institutes of Health, June 5, 2009. http://ghr.nlm.nih.gov.
18. Bruce Steiger and Rick Karl, "Krystie's Story," Cure Tay-Sachs Foundation, September 2007. www.curetay-sachs.org.
19. Jeff Alexander, "3-Year-Old Liam Hoekstra Makes a Very Strong Impression," *Muskegon* (MI) *Chronicle*, January 1, 2009. www.mlive.com.

How Should Genetic Test Results Be Used?

20. Quoted in Deborah Franklin, "Family Struggles with Ambiguity of Genetic Testing," National Public Radio, December 30, 2008. www.npr.org.
21. Amy Harmon, "Facing Life with a Lethal Gene," *New York Times*, March 18, 2007. www.nytimes.com.
22. Rahul K. Parikh, "Sarah Palin's Choice," *Salon*, September 5, 2008. www.salon.com.
23. Quoted in Devon Williams, "Doctors Advised Abortion; Baby Born Healthy," Citizen Link, February 25, 2008. www.citizenlink.org.

24. Quoted in *New York Daily News*, "'Cancer-Free' Baby Born in London Amid Controversy over Genetic Testing," January 9, 2009. www.nydaily news.com.

25. BreastCancer.org, "Deciding Who in the Family Should Get Tested," March 18, 2009. www.breastcancer.org.

26. Peta Bee, "Can a DNA Test Show Whether Your Child Will Be a Sporting Star?" *Times* (London), January 5, 2009. www.timesonline.co.uk.

Can Genetic Disorders Be Cured?

27. Quoted in Elaine Schmidt, "Drug Reverses Mental Retardation Caused by Genetic Disorder," UCLA Newsroom, June 22, 2008. www.newsroom.ucla. edu.

28. Darlene Davis, interviewed by Devon Williams, "Friday Five: Darlene Davis," CitizenLink, May 28, 2008. www. citizenlink.org.

29. Quoted in the Denver Channel, "Stem Cells Save Two Brothers with Skin Disease," March 3, 2008. www.thedenver channel.com.

30. Quoted in Elizabeth Flores, "Long-Shot Stem-Cell Treatment Gives Two Brothers a Future," *Minneapolis Star Tribune*, June 3, 2008. www.startri bune.com.

31. Genetics Home Reference, "Gene Therapy," National Institutes of Health, June 5, 2009. http://ghr.nlm.nih.gov.

32. Quoted in BBC News, "Nano-treatment to Torpedo Cancer," March 10, 2009. http://news.bbc.co.uk.

33. Quoted in April Frawley Birdwell, "UF Makes Gene Therapy Breakthrough in Treating Severe Genetic Disorder," University of Florida News, May 28, 2009. http://news.ufl.edu.

34. Mark Henderson, "Daily Pill to Beat Genetic Diseases," *Times* (London), April 23, 2007. www.timesonline.co.uk.

List of Illustrations

Index